Manual on
IMAGING IN OBSTETRICS AND GYNECOLOGY

AF729939

Manual on IMAGING IN OBSTETRICS AND GYNECOLOGY

Series Editors

Nandita Palshetkar
MD FCPS FICOG FRCOG (UK)
Professor Emeritus
Department of Obstetrics and Gynecology
DY Patil School of Medicine
Navi Mumbai, Maharashtra, India
Founder and Medical Director of the
Famous Bloom IVF Group

Hrishikesh D Pai
MD FRCOG (UK-HON) FCPS FICOG MSc (USA)
Trustee, FIGO, Asia Oceania (2023–25)
Professor, DY Patil University
Navi Mumbai, Maharashtra, India
Immediate Past President FOGSI (2022–23)
Founder and Medical Director
Bloom IVF Group, Mumbai

Niranjan Chavan
MD FICOG FCPS DGO DFP MICOG DICOG Diploma in Endoscopy (USA)
Professor and Unit Chief
Department of Obstetrics and Gynecology
Lokmanya Tilak Medical College and General Hospital
Mumbai, Maharashtra, India

Editors

Bela Bhatt
MBBS MD (Obs & Gyne) FICOG
Lead Consultant
Dr Bela's Women's Hospital and
Fetal Medicine Center, Mumbai
Fetal Medicine Consultant
Dr Babasaheb Ambedkar Memorial
Central Railway Hospital
Mumbai, Maharashtra, India
Chairperson
FOGSI Imaging Science Committee
Treasurer, Association of Fellow
Gynaecologists, Mumbai
Managing Council Member, ISPAT
FOGSI National Talent Co-Ordinator
(2019–20 and 2022–23)

Chinmayee Ratha
MS (Obs & Gyne) FRCOG (UK) FICOG FIMSA
Diploma in Fetal Medicine (FMF-UK)
Director
Resolution Centre of Fetal Medicine
Hyderabad
Lead Consultant Fetal Medicine
KIMS Sunshine Hospitals, KIMS Cuddles
Kondapur, Hyderabad
Visiting Consultant
Arete Hospitals, Gachibowli
Hyderabad, Telangana, India
Chairperson
FOGSI Perinatology Committee
Centre Head ICOG Fetal Medicine
Certification Course

Co-Editors

**Neena Malhotra, Narendra Malhotra,
Parag Biniwale, Ritu Hinduja, Tejal Poddar**

JAYPEE

JAYPEE BROTHERS MEDICAL PUBLISHERS
The Health Sciences Publisher
New Delhi | London

Message from Series Editors

Dear AICOG 2025 delegates,

It is a matter of great pride that the landmark AICOG 2025 is being held in the city of Mumbai, Maharashtra, India. The Organizing Committee and the hosts Mumbai Obstetric and Gynaecological Society have left no stone unturned in their quest to make this a historic event by aiming to have a scientific program of the highest caliber, punctuated by fantastic keynotes and orations, graced by the best international faculty in the field of Obstetrics, Gynecology and its subspecialities along with a cultural treat every evening to cater to the audience which hails from far-flung corners of India and the globe.

On this occasion, the academic stalwarts and senior FOGSIans have burned the midnight oil at both ends to contribute and create a set of AICOG 2025 Workshop Manuals that aim to amalgamate the most recent scientific advancements and evidence-based best practices in a nutshell for the delegates to take home and implement in their practices when they have returned from this magnificent event.

We acknowledge the efforts of all the editors, co-editors, authors, co-authors, co-contributors and junior authors who have sometimes worked at short notice to submit excellent chapters and articles included in the final publication. We also wish to take this opportunity to thank Shri Jitendar P Vij (Group Chairman) and Mr Ankit Vij (Managing Director) of M/s Jaypee Brothers Medical Publishers (P) Ltd, New Delhi, India, in publishing the book and their associates, particularly Ms Chetna Malhotra (Senior Director—Professional Publishing, Marketing, and Business Development), Ms Kritika Dua (Senior Commissiong Editor), and Mr Priyansh Saxena (Development Editor), who have been prompt, efficient, and most helpful.

We hope that the delegates and the attendees will enjoy reading this publication and the scientific data included therein will help to shape your knowledge, attitudes and practices and ultimately benefit the women of our country, whom we all serve.

Nandita Palshetkar
Organizing Chairperson, AICOG Mumbai, 2025

Hrishikesh D Pai
Chairperson, Scientific Committee, AICOG Mumbai, 2025

Niranjan Chavan
Organizing Secretary, AICOG Mumbai, 2025

FOGSI

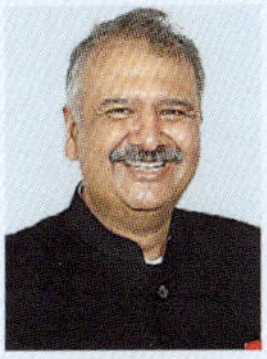

Jaydeep Tank
President 2024–2025

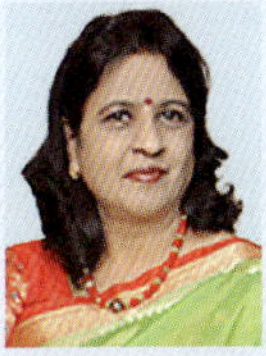

Madhuri Patel
Secretary General

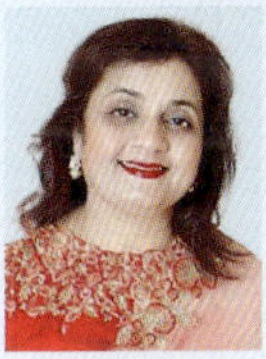

Sunita Tandulwadkar
President 2025–2026

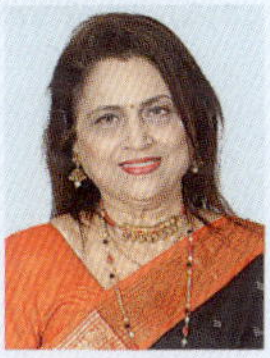

Suvarna Khadilkar
Deputy Secretary General

AICOG 2025 Core Committee

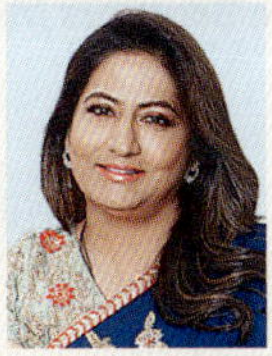

Nandita Palshetkar
Organizing Chairperson

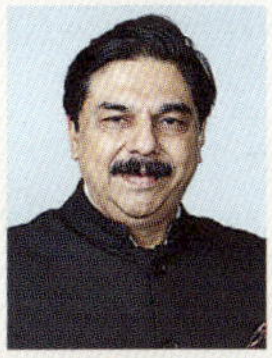

Hrishikesh D Pai
Chairperson, Scientific Committee

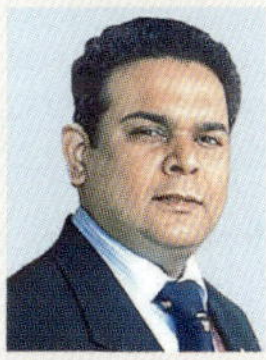

Niranjan Chavan
Organizing Secretary

Editors

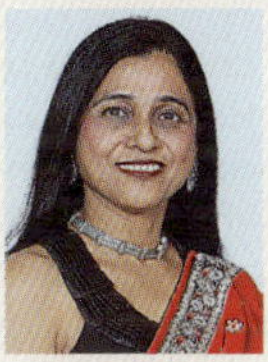

Bela Bhatt

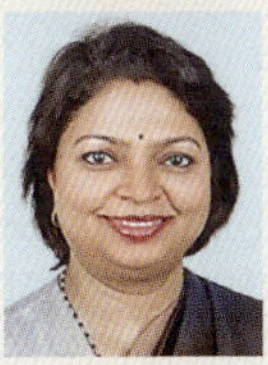

Chinmayee Ratha

Vice Chairpersons

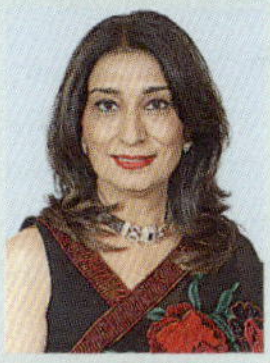

Rishma Dhillon Pai

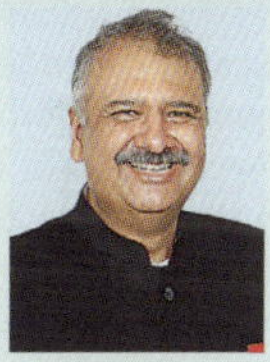

Jaydeep Tank

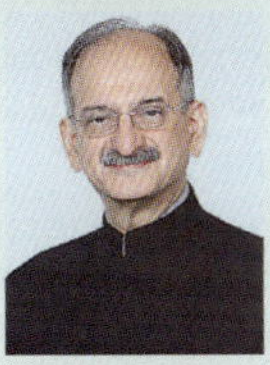

Nozer Sheriar

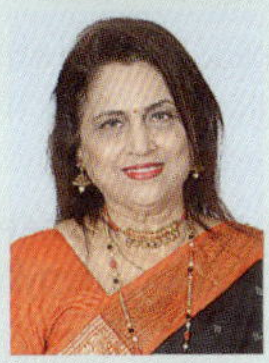

Suvarna Khadilkar

AICOG 2025 Publication Committee

Pratik Tambe	Rohan Palshetkar
Pradnya Supe	Manan Boob

JAYPEE Jaypee Brothers Medical Publishers (P) Ltd

Headquarters
Jaypee Brothers Medical Publishers (P) Ltd
EMCA House, 23/23-B
Ansari Road, Daryaganj
New Delhi 110 002, India
Landline: +91-11-23272143, +91-11-23272703
+91-11-23282021, +91-11-23245672
Email: jaypee@jaypeebrothers.com

Corporate Office
Jaypee Brothers Medical Publishers (P) Ltd
4838/24, Ansari Road, Daryaganj
New Delhi 110 002, India
Phone: +91-11-43574357
Fax: +91-11-43574314
Email: jaypee@jaypeebrothers.com

Overseas Office
JP Medical Ltd.
83, Victoria Street, London
SW1H 0HW (UK)
Phone: +44 20 3170 8910
Fax: +44 (0)20 3008 6180
Email: info@jpmedpub.com

Website: www.jaypeebrothers.com
Website: www.jaypeedigital.com

Inquiries for bulk sales may be solicited at: jaypee@jaypeebrothers.com

Manual on Imaging in Obstetrics and Gynecology

First Edition: **2025**

ISBN: 978-93-6616-864-7

Printed at: Samrat Offset Pvt. Ltd.

Contributors

Aditi Shastri
MBBS DNB (Obs & Gyne) Fellowship in Fetal Medicine
Consultant
Resolution Centre of Fetal Medicine
Hyderabad, Telangana, India

Bharani Vijayaragavan
MBBS DGO DNB
Senior Resident
Sri Ramachandra Institute of Health and Research
Chennai, Tamil Nadu, India

Chanchal Singh
MBBS MD (Obs & Gyne) MRCOG (UK) Fellow Maternal Fetal Medicine, Fetal Medicine Foundation Certified (NUH, Singapore)
Lead Consultant
Fetal Medicine
Department of Fetal Medicine
Madhukar Rainbow
Children's Hospital and
BirthRight, by Rainbow Hospitals
New Delhi, India

Chandrakant Garg
MBBS DGO Fellowship in Fetal Medicine
Fetal Medicine Consultant
Jaipur Fetal Medicine and Research Center
Jaipur, Rajasthan, India

Debasmita Mandal
MBBS MD FICOG FIAOG Post-Doctoral Fellowship in Fetal Medicine
Chief Fetal Medicine Consultant
Krishnaya Institute of
Cardiac and Fetal Sciences
NRS Medical College
Kolkata, West Bengal, India

Devanshi Mishra MBBS MD
Associate Consultant
Department of Reproductive Medicine
Bansal Hospital
Bhopal, Madhya Pradesh, India

Karra Sahithi Reddy
MBBS DGO Fellow Fetal Medicine (FMF and ICOG Accredited)
Consultant
Resolution Centre of Fetal Medicine
Hyderabad, Telangana, India

Karthik Senthivel
MBBS MDRD PDF Advanced University Certificate in Maternal-Fetal Medicine (Fetal Medicine Barcelona) FMF UK Certified for Fetal Interventions Clinical Genetics Fellowship (NIMS)
Clinical Head
Karu Fetal Diagnosis, Therapy
Genetics and Research Institute
Trichy, Tamil Nadu, India

Malvika Jain MBBS MS
Senior Resident
Sri Ramachandra Institute of Health and Research
Chennai, Tamil Nadu, India

Prasanna Roy MBBS MS
Fetal Medicine Consultant
Ultra Clinic
Asansol, West Bengal, India

Priya Bhave Chittawar MBBS MD
Head
Department of Reproductive Medicine
Bansal Hospital
Bhopal, Madhya Pradesh, India

Smita Dhengle
MBBS DGO DNB MNAMS FICOG Fellowship in Fetal Medicine
Consultant Fetal Medicine
Bansal Hospital
Bhopal, Madhya Pradesh, India

Uttara Gupta MBBS
Senior Resident
Department of Reproductive Medicine
Bansal Hospital
Bhopal, Madhya Pradesh, India

Vrunda Appannagari
MBBS DNB MRCOG
Senior Consultant
Fetal Medicine
Department of Fetal Medicine
Madhukar Rainbow Children's Hospital and BirthRight, by Rainbow Hospitals
New Delhi, India

Preface

The *Manual on Imaging in Obstetrics and Gynecology* by FOGSI features 10 comprehensive chapters that's through light on the basics of imaging in obstetrics and gynecology.

The authors have spent their valuable time to share their knowledge on various topics like ultrasound in PAS, first trimester anomalies, basics of obstetric Doppler, late onset anomalies, soft markers, mid-trimester structural anomalies, intrapartum USG, cervical length, liqour assessment, and also ultrasound in adnexal masses. This will surely be of great use to all the obstetricians and gynecologists in their daily practice. We are extremely thankful to all the authors for the same. We are equally grateful to our leaders of FOGSI Dr Hrishikesh D Pai, Dr Nandita Palshetkar, Dr Niranjan Chavan and Dr Rohan Palshetkar for giving us the opportunity.

Our sincere thanks to Shri Jitendar P Vij (Group Chairman) and Mr Ankit Vij (Managing Director) of M/s Jaypee Brothers Medical Publishers (P) Ltd New Delhi, India for their support, encouragement and logistics. We express our special thanks to the entire production team of M/s Jaypee Brothers Medical Publishers (P) Ltd, especially Mr Priyansh Saxena (Development Editor) for their hard work, professionalism and for helping us throughout the journey of this publication.

May the manual be a guiding light to serve as a invaluable resources in understanding the intricacies of vaginal surgeries for our practitioners and academicians.

Enjoy Reading!!

Series Editors: Nandita Palshetkar, Hrishikesh D Pai, Niranjan Chavan
Editors: Bela Bhatt, Chinmayee Ratha
Co-Editors: Neena Malhotra, Narendra Malhotra, Parag Biniwale, Ritu Hinduja, Tejal Poddar

Contents

1 CHAPTER

Placenta Accreta Spectrum

Smita Dhengle

Placenta accreta is a serious obstetric complication characterized by the abnormal adherence of the placenta to the uterine wall. This condition can lead to significant maternal morbidity and mortality due to complications such as severe hemorrhage, infection, and the need for surgical interventions like hysterectomy. The prevalence of placenta accreta has been rising, primarily due to increased cesarean delivery rates, with estimates suggesting it occurs at approximately 1 in 533 pregnancies.

NORMAL PLACENTA

It is made of two layers: Decidua and superficial myometrium, the decidua containing the tip of the spiral arteries and the superficial myometrium containing the spiral and basal arteries.

In normal placentation, there is hypoechoic retroplacental space known as *Clear Zone*.

The appearance of the clear zone changes with advancing gestational age, location of placenta in the uterine cavity and direct pressure by the ultrasound probe **(Fig. 1)**.

Uterine Scar

Muscles including myometrium do not heal by regenerating muscle fiber leading to collagen + myofiber disarray, tissue edema, inflammation and elastosis.

Scar tissue is thinner and less elastic and more prone to injury than the intact muscle therefore lower uterine segment is thinner and contains less muscle fiber leading to C section scar defect.

Placenta Accreta Spectrum

It is the failure of normal decidualization in an area of a previous uterine scar.

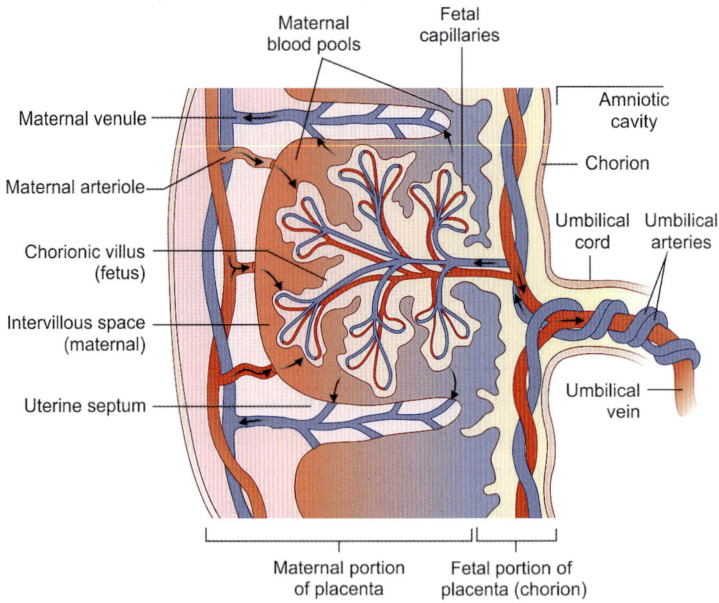

Fig. 1: Blood vein system of placenta.

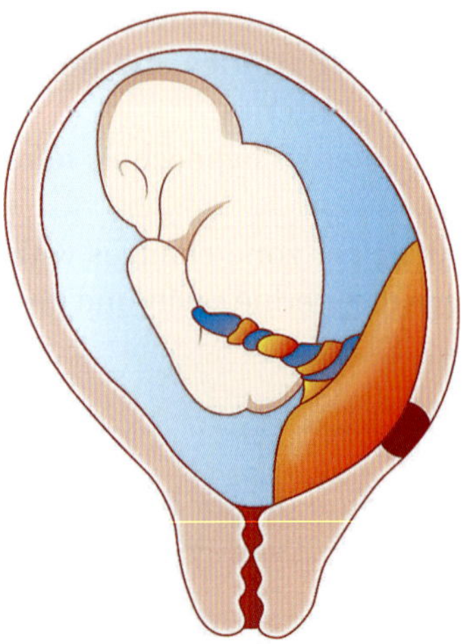

Fig. 2: Placenta accreta.

There are three main types of placenta accreta, classified based on the depth of placental invasion:

1. *Placenta accreta:* The placenta attaches deeply to the uterine wall but does not penetrate the muscle **(Fig. 2)**.
2. *Placenta increta:* The placenta invades the myometrium (muscle layer of the uterus) **(Fig. 3)**.

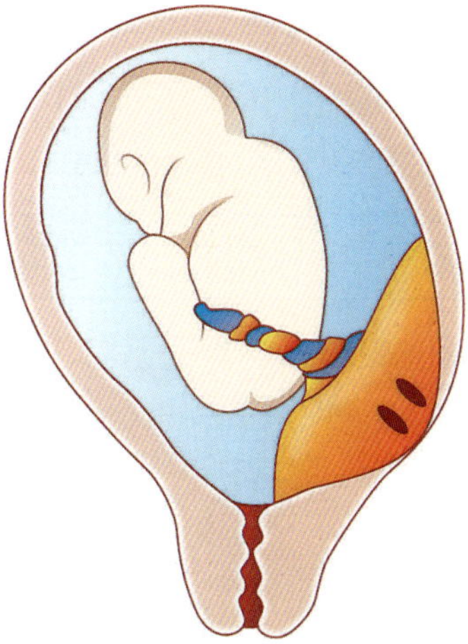

Fig. 3: Placenta increta.

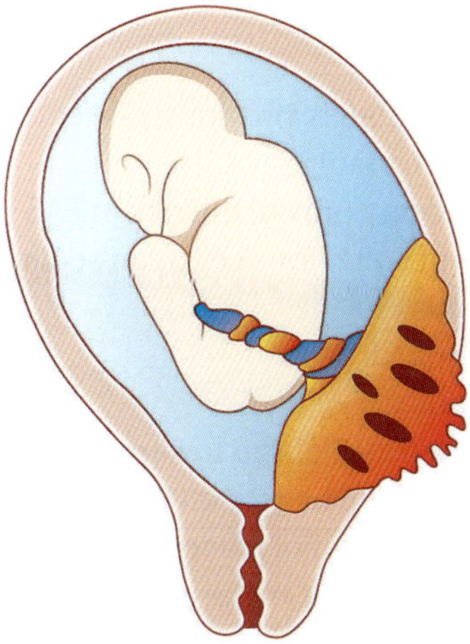

Fig. 4: Placenta percreta.

3. *Placenta percreta:* The placenta penetrates through the uterine wall and may attach to adjacent organs, such as the bladder **(Fig. 4)**.

PAS disorder may coexist within same placenta **(Fig. 5)**.

RISK FACTORS

Several factors increase the risk of developing placenta accreta:

Direct Surgical Scar

- Surgical termination of pregnancy
- Dilatation and curettage

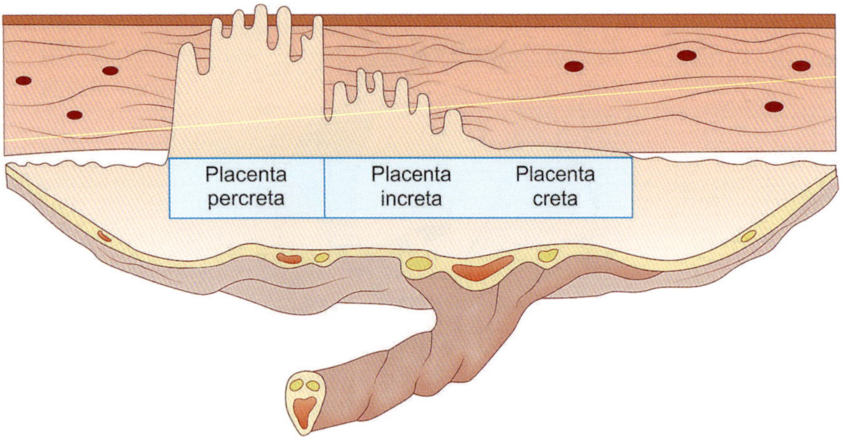

Fig. 5: PAS disorder in same placenta.

- Myomectomy
- Endometrial resection
- Previous cesarean section
- The main risk factor for PAS is previous C-section delivery and placenta previa in the current pregnancy
- In the presence of placenta previa, the risk of PAS increases:
    - 3% in those without a previous cesarean section
    - 10% after 1 previous CS
    - 40% after 2 previous CS
    - 60% after 3 previous CS
    - Scar in the myometrium of the lower uterine segment—encourages both implantation of the blastocyst in the area of the scar and abnormal adherence or invasion of placental villi within the scar tissue.

Poor vascularization and tissue oxygenation in the area of a cesarean scar is associated with local failure of re-epithelialization and decidualization and has an impact on both implantation and placentation.

Nonsurgical Scar

- Uterine artery embolization
- Endometritis
- Chemotherapy and radiation
- Intrauterine devices
- Asherman syndrome

Uterine Anomaly

- Bicornuate uterus
- Adenomyosis
- Myotonic dystrophy

DIAGNOSIS

Placenta Accreta Spectrum: Ultrasound Signs

Loss of the Clear Zone

In this hypoechoic retroplacental zone is not visible it is found in about 70% of cases **(Fig. 6)**

Myometrial Thinning

The myometrium under the placenta measures <1 mm or becomes undetectable **(Fig. 7)**.

This sign is found in about 50% of affected cases and *not a strong ultrasound marker for PAS.*

Scar dehiscence: The myometrium can become so thin that the placenta can be seen through it at delivery **(Fig. 8)**.

Uterine window represents deficient myometrium rather than abnormal placentation. The placental bladder border is smooth and regular.

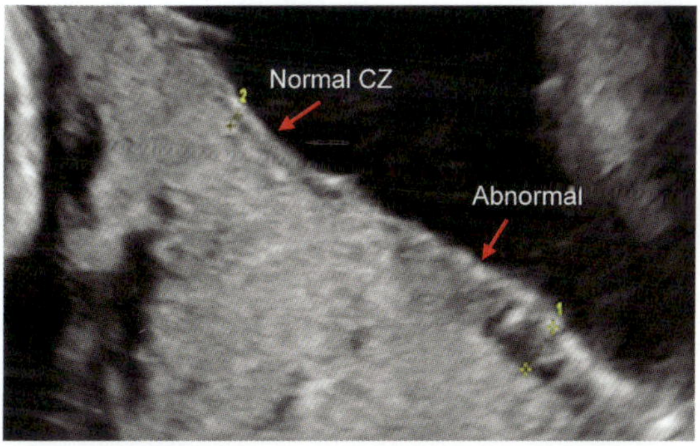

Fig. 6: Hypoechoic retroplacental zone.

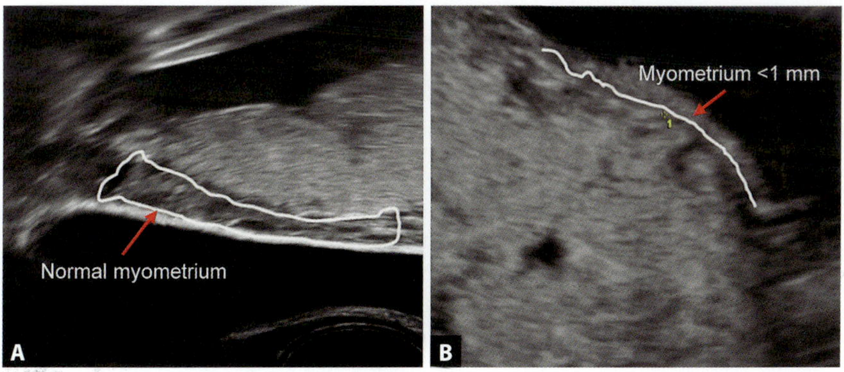

Figs. 7A and B: (A) Normal myometrium; (B) Myometrium <1 mm.

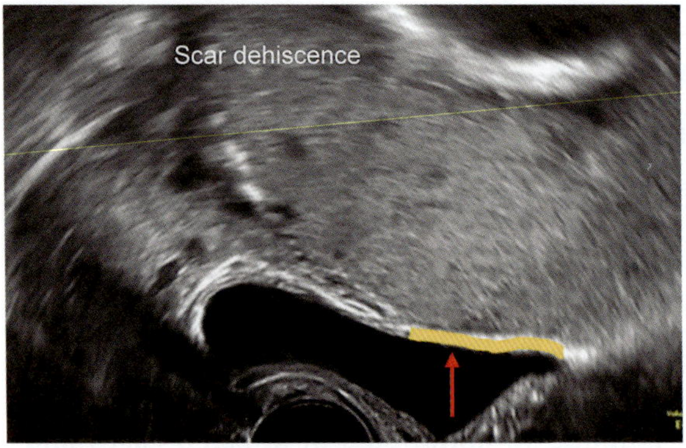

Fig. 8: Scar dehiscence.

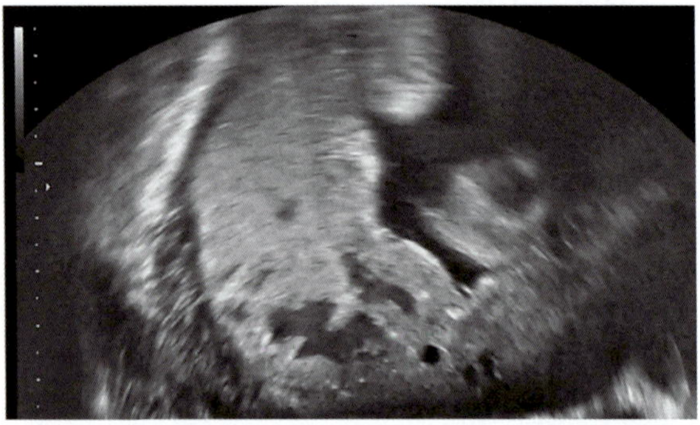

Fig. 9: Placental lacunae.

TABLE 1: Placental lacunae vs. lakes.

Lacunae	*Lakes*
Irregular margins	Regular margins
Numerous	Fewer
Feeder vessel commonly seen	Feeder vessel uncommonly seen
High velocity blood vessel seen	

Placental Lacunae

- It is the most common ultrasound sign in PAS **(Fig. 9)**. It is formed due to distorted cotyledons and interlobular septa.
- Lacunae have direct high velocity maternal blood from a radial or arcuate artery, the peak systolic velocity is often >10 cm/sec. Their shape is not influenced by the filling of the bladder or pressure from the probe.

Table 1 shows the difference between lacunae and lakes.

Bladder Wall Interruption

It is the irregularity of the bladder wall between the placenta and the bladder due to massive developing of dilated vessels between the anterior uterine wall and the posterior bladder wall.

Placental Bulge

Placental bulge represents villous invasion deep into the myometrium distorting the uterine shape, the placenta bulges into the surrounding tissue, usually the bladder **(Fig. 10)**.

Exophytic Mass

- Seen only in the case of placenta percreta **(Fig. 11)**
- It is the invasion of placental tissue through the myometrium into extrauterine organs.

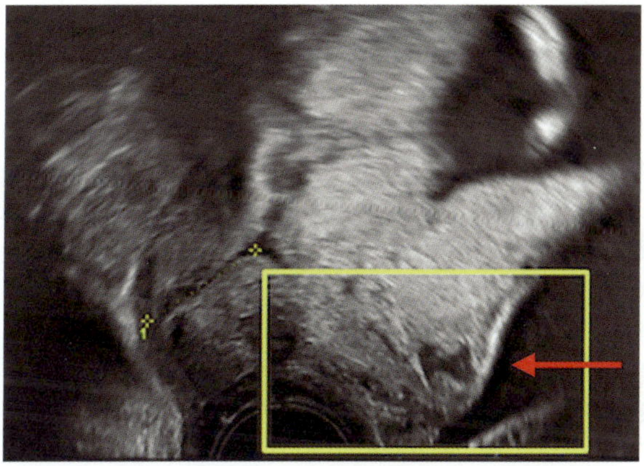

Fig. 10: Placental bulge.

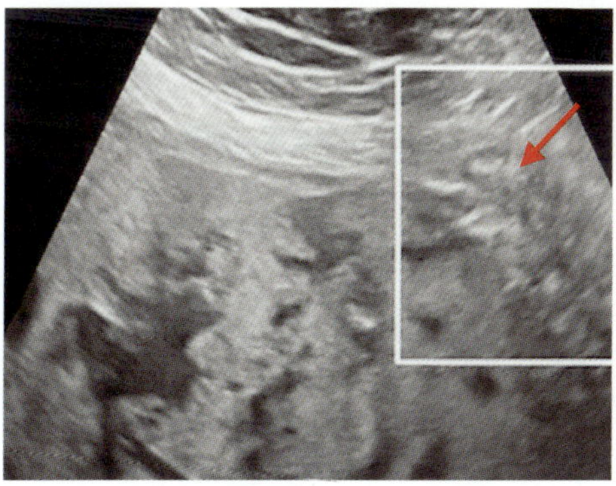

Fig. 11: Exophytic mass.

Uterovesical Hypervascularity and Bridging Vessels

These are actually dilated vessels within the peritoneum between the bladder and uterus and these vessels do not cross the uterine serosa or penetrate the bladder wall **(Fig. 12)**. Color Doppler signals arising in the myometrium and crossing the uterine wall into the bladder. This is not evidence of placenta percreta. Hypervascularization within or under the placental bed is found in about 80% of cases of placenta increta and 75% result from excessive dilatation of the cases of placenta percreta.

Subplacental Hypervascularity

Characterized by abnormal subplacental blood flow.

Lacunae Feeder Vessels

These feeder vessels are often seen entering placental lacunae with high velocity blood flows arising directly from a radial or arcuate artery.

MRI

- Excellent tool for diagnosing the PAS.
- Placental bulge and uterine serosal hypervascularity are useful MRI features for differentiating placenta percreta and increta from placenta accreta **(Fig. 13)**.
  - The more extensive and invasive the placenta, the more distorted the vascular architecture should be.
  - Marked heterogeneity and intraplacental dark bands in a T2-weighted image are the most sensitive MRI signs for detecting PAS.
  - In cases with the absence of placental heterogeneity or dark intraplacental banding, evaluation of the uterine contour and myometrial changes may be helpful for diagnosing PAS.
  - The presence of two or more MRI features increases the reliability of a PAS diagnosis.

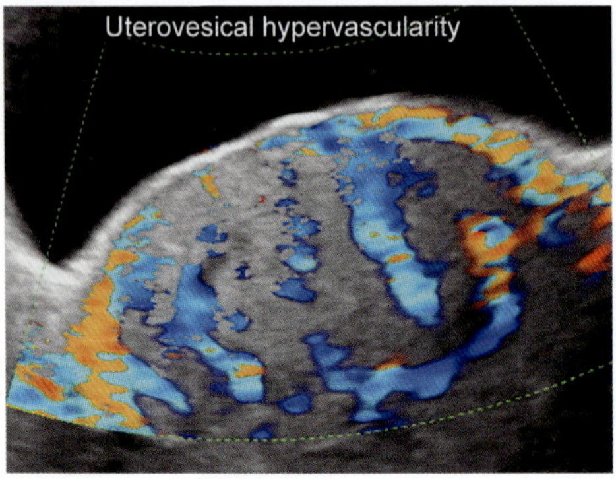

Fig. 12: Uterovesical hypervascularity.

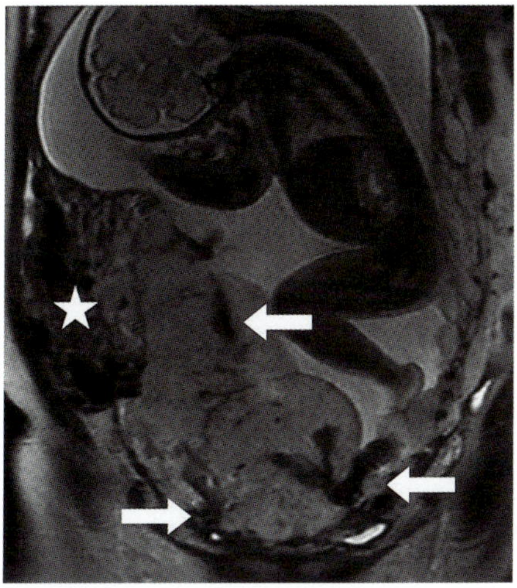

Fig. 13: MRI of placenta percreta.

- Regarding the bladder tenting sign, under- or overdistension of the bladder may cause a false interpretation of this sign.
- Some imaging planes can lead to a false-positive diagnosis of PAS due to the curved shape of the uterus. Suspicious findings should be confirmed in more than one imaging plane.
- MRI should not be used alone. A combined study that includes both MRI and US, in addition to the clinical context, must be performed.

MANAGEMENT STRATEGIES

Management of placenta accreta involves a multidisciplinary approach, often requiring careful planning and coordination among obstetricians, anesthesiologists, and surgical teams including interventional radiologists. The primary treatment options include:

- *Cesarean hysterectomy:* This is the most common approach, where the uterus is removed after the delivery of the fetus. This method minimizes the risk of severe hemorrhages that can occur if attempts are made to remove the placenta.
- *Conservative management:* In select cases, particularly when there is a desire to preserve fertility, conservative management may be considered. This approach can include leaving the placenta in situ and monitoring the patient closely, with interventions such as methotrexate or uterine artery embolization. Prophylactic transcatheter uterine artery embolization after the baby is delivered is also being followed.
- *Postpartum care:* Women diagnosed with placenta accreta require close monitoring postpartum due to the risk of hemorrhage and infection. If the placenta is retained, management may involve medication or surgical intervention to address complications.

CONCLUSION

Placenta accreta is a complex and increasingly common condition that poses significant risks to maternal health. Early diagnosis and a well-coordinated management plan are essential to improve outcomes for both mother and child. As the rates of cesarean deliveries continue to rise, awareness and understanding of placenta accreta will be crucial for healthcare providers to ensure the safety and well-being of affected patients.

SUGGESTED READING

1. Cali G, Forlani F, Less C, et al. Prenatal ultrasound staging system for placenta accreta spectrum disorders. Ultrasound Obstet Gynecol. 2019;53(6):752-60. doi: 10.1002/uog.20246. Epub 2019 May 6.
2. https://www.acog.org/clinical/clinical-guidance/obstetric-care-consensus/articles/2018/12/placenta-accreta-spectrum.
3. Sitthipong S, Patcharin P, Sirikan B. Magnetic resonance imaging of placenta accreta spectrum: a step-by-step approach. Korean J Radiol. 2020.

2 CHAPTER

Ultrasonographic Evaluation of Adnexal Masses

Priya Bhave Chittawar, Devanshi Mishra, Uttara Gupta

BACKGROUND

An adnexal mass (mass of the ovary, fallopian tube, or surrounding connective tissues) is a common gynecologic issue and may present with pelvic pain or pressure or be an incidental finding on pelvic examination or pelvic imaging. It may come from functional or physiological changes, inflammatory processes, endometriosis, benign and malignant tumors.

The overall incidence of a symptomatic ovarian cyst in a premenopausal female being malignant is approximately 1:1000 increasing to 3:1000 at the age of 50.[1] Being common in postmenopausal women as well, the exact prevalence is unknown due to limited amount of published data. However, estimated incidence to be anywhere between 5 and 17%.[2]

ASSESSMENT OF ADNEXAL MASSES

A thorough medical history should be taken from patients with specific attention to risk factors for ovarian malignancy and a family history of ovarian or breast cancer. Other factors to consider are symptoms of pelvic pain (adnexal torsion or endometriosis, pelvic inflammatory disease, or an acutely hemorrhagic corpus luteum cyst), abdominal distention accompanied by gastrointestinal complaints and weight loss (advanced ovarian malignancy) and use of hormonal contraception (which may affect the likelihood of functional ovarian cysts).[3]

Along with history and physical examination basic blood work-up to be done with special attention to tumor markers. CA-125 can be used for primary evaluation, as it allows the Risk of Malignancy Index (RMI) of ovarian cysts in postmenopausal women. Other markers such as human epididymis protein 4 (HE4), carcinoembryonic antigen (CEA), cancer antigen 19-9 (CA19-9), alpha-fetoprotein, lactate dehydrogenase (LDH) or beta-human chorionic gonadotropin are also assessed for evaluation of ovarian cysts.[2]

ROLE OF ULTRASOUND IN EVALUATION

With advancements in transvaginal ultrasonography (TVS) techniques, precision of diagnosing adnexal masses has increased multi-folds. The size and composition of the mass (cystic, solid, or mixed), its laterality, as well as the presence or absence of septations, mural nodules, papillary excrescences, or free fluid in the pelvis, should be assessed through TVS. For the evaluation of vascular features of lesions in the pelvis, spectral, color Doppler ultrasound can be helpful.[4]

Scope of TVS in evaluating adnexal masses, is increasing and, in expert hands, it might be as informative as magnetic resonance imaging. Hence, understanding the basics of TVS and learning the latest classifications has become important.

INTERNATIONAL OVARIAN TUMOR ANALYSIS (IOTA)

The IOTA Simple Rules consist of five ultrasound features suggestive of malignancy (M-features) and five features suggestive of benignity (B-features). Based on the presence or absence of these features, an adnexal mass can be classified as benign, malignant, or indeterminate.[5]

IOTA Simple Rules

The International Ovarian Tumor Analysis (IOTA) rules for benign and malignant are described in **Table 1**.[6]

Applications of IOTA Simple Rules

- *Benign mass:* If one or more B-features are present without any M-features, the mass is considered likely benign.
- *Malignant mass:* If one or more M-features are present without any B-features, the mass is considered likely malignant.
- *Inconclusive:* If both M-features and B-features are present or if no features are present, the mass is classified as indeterminate, warranting further evaluation.

The IOTA ADNEX Model

The IOTA ADNEX model (Assessment of Different NEoplasias in the adneXa) is a multivariate risk prediction model designed to estimate the risk of

TABLE 1: IOTA rules for benign and malignant.

Benign (B-rules)	*Malignant (M-rules)*
Unilocular cysts	Irregular solid tumor
Presence of solid components where the largest solid component <0.7 cm	Ascites
Presence of acoustic shadowing	At least four papillary structures
Smooth multilocular tumor with largest diameter <10 cm	Irregular multilocular solid tumor with largest diameter >10 cm
No blood flow	Very good blood flow

(IOTA: international ovarian tumor analysis)

TABLE 2: ADNEX model parameters and description.

Parameter	*Description*
Age	Age of the patient in years
CA-125 level	Serum CA-125 level in IU/mL (optional but improves accuracy)
Type of center	Whether the ultrasound is performed at an oncology center
Maximal diameter of the mass	Largest diameter of the mass in millimeters (mm)
Presence of solid component	Presence or absence of a solid component within the mass
Number of papillary projections	Count of papillary projections in the cyst
Presence of acoustic shadows	Presence or absence of acoustic shadows on ultrasound
Ascites	Presence or absence of free fluid in the pelvis or abdomen
Irregular internal cyst walls	Smooth vs. irregular inner walls of the cyst

malignancy in adnexal masses. Unlike the Simple Rules, the ADNEX model provides a risk percentage for four different types of ovarian neoplasms:

- Benign tumor
- Borderline tumor
- Stage I—Invasive ovarian cancer
- Stage II–IV—Invasive ovarian cancer or secondary metastatic tumor

Parameters Used in the ADNEX Model

The ADNEX model uses a combination of clinical and ultrasound variables **(Table 2)**.

The model uses these parameters to generate a risk score for each type of neoplasm, helping guide further management and referral decisions.

OVARIAN-ADNEXAL REPORTING AND DATA SYSTEM (O-RADS)

The *Ovarian-Adnexal Reporting and Data System (O-RADS)* is a standardized reporting system developed by the American College of Radiology (ACR), in 2018, to evaluate adnexal masses using ultrasound. The system categorizes adnexal masses based on their ultrasonographic appearance, clinical context, and associated risk of malignancy and function as guidance in the management of average-risk patients without acute symptoms who demonstrate adnexal lesions.[7]

TABLE 3: O-RADS scoring.

O-RADS scoring	*Category*	*Risk of malignancy (percentage)*	*Ultrasound findings*	*Management*
O-RADS0	Incomplete evaluation	–	Incomplete or non-diagnostic ultrasound	Repeat ultrasound/ alternate imaging study such as MRI
O-RADS1	Normal findings	0	Normal ovaries or physiological cysts (e.g., follicular cysts)	No additional imaging or imaging follow-up is necessary
O-RADS2	Almost certainly benign	<1	Simple cysts, hemorrhagic cysts, dermoid cysts, endometriomas	Follow-up if symptomatic or as per guidelines
O-RADS3	Low risk of malignancy	1–<10	Unilocular cysts with one thin septation or mild solid components	Follow-up ultrasound or referral
O-RADS4	Intermediate risk of malignancy	10–50	Multilocular cysts, solid components with irregular walls	Referral to a gynecologic oncologist
O-RADS5	High risk of malignancy	>50	Solid masses, thick septations, papillary projections, ascites	Urgent referral to gynecologic oncologist

(O-RADS: Ovarian-Adnexal Reporting and Data System)

O-RADS provides a scoring system ranging from 0 to 5, based on the risk of malignancy associated with different ultrasound features **(Table 3)**.

Detailed Explanation of O-RADS Categories

1. *O-RADS0—Incomplete evaluation:* Ultrasound examination is incomplete, common reasons include poor image quality, patient discomfort, or obscured visualization due to bowel gas or obesity.
2. *O-RADS1—Normal findings:* Masses in this category have a 0% risk of malignancy. This suggests normal premenopausal ovary.
   - *Follicle:* Uniocular, anechoic cyst (≤3 cm) **(Fig. 1)**
   - *Corpus luteum:* Thick-walled cyst (≤3 cm) ± crenulated inner margins, internal echoes, peripheral flow or hypoechoic region with peripheral flow but without characteristic cystic component **(Fig. 2)**.
3. *O-RADS2—Almost certainly benign:* Masses in this category have a <1% risk of malignancy and include:
   - *Simple cysts:* Anechoic, thin-walled, unilocular cysts without solid components, >3 cm–<10 cm in premenopausal, <10 cm in postmenopausal.

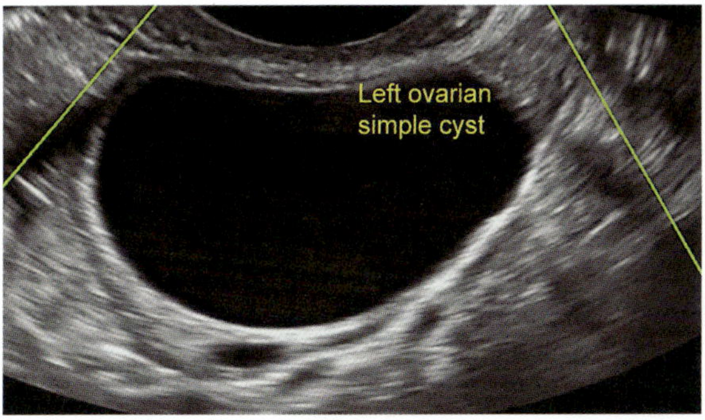

Fig. 1: Follicle.

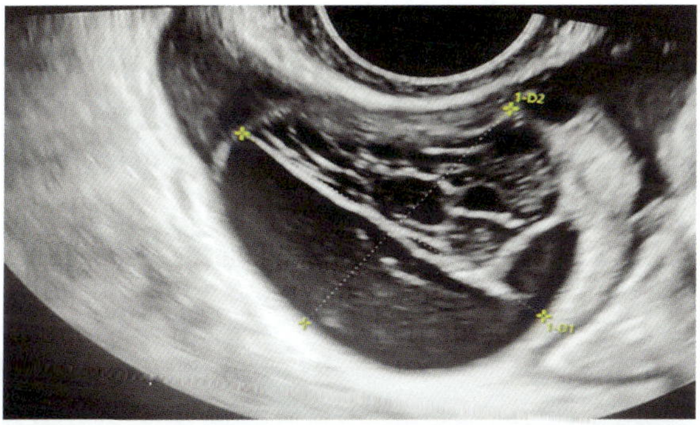

Fig. 2: Corpus luteum.

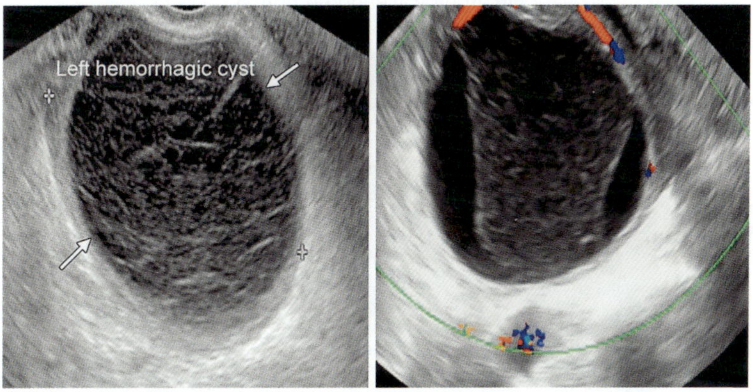

Fig. 3: Typical hemorrhagic cysts.

- *Typical hemorrhagic cysts (<10 cm):* Cysts with fibrin strands or a "lace-like" appearance, reticular pattern, or retracting clot **(Fig. 3)**.
- *Typical dermoid cysts (mature cystic teratomas) (<10 cm):* Complex cysts with echogenic foci (e.g., hair, calcifications), hyperechoic lines and dots, floating echogenic structures **(Fig. 4)**.

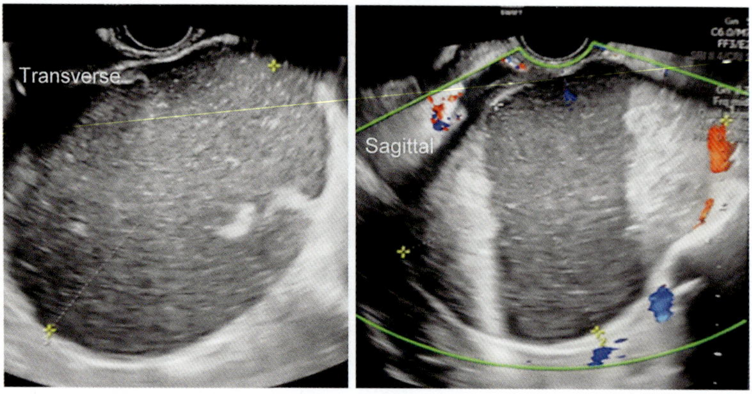

Fig. 4: Typical dermoid cysts.

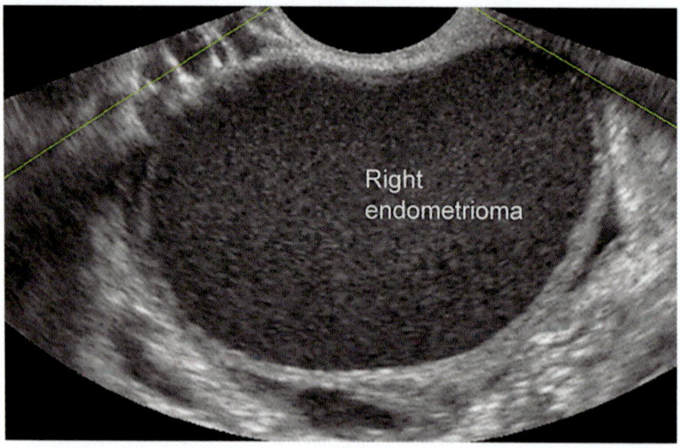

Fig. 5: Typical endometriomas.

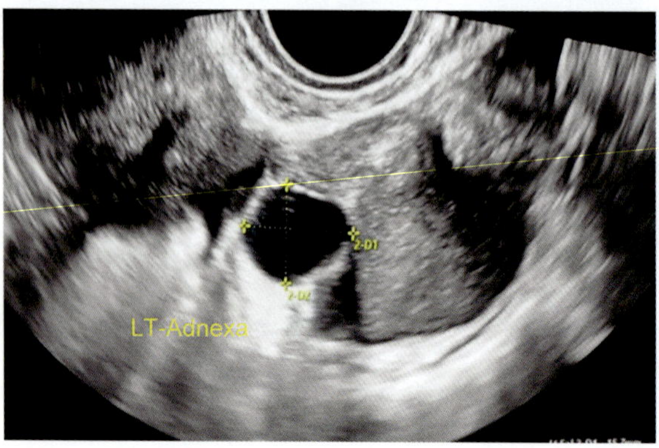

Fig. 6: Simple paraovarian cyst.

- *Typical endometriomas (<10 cm):* Homogeneous, hypoechoic cysts with diffuse low-level echoes, often described as "ground-glass" appearance **(Fig. 5)**.
- Simple paraovarian cyst (any size) **(Fig. 6)**

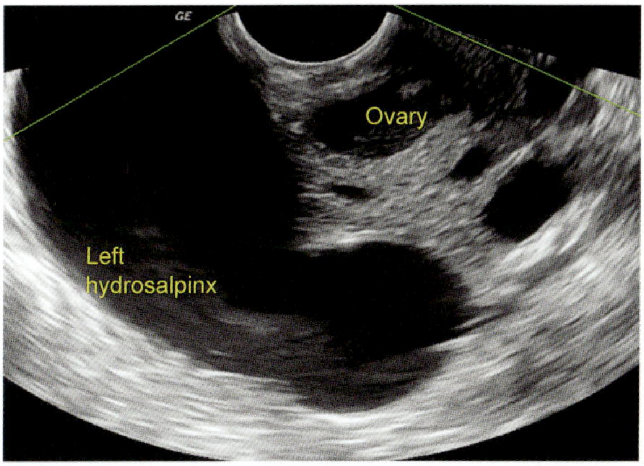

Fig. 7: Typical hydrosalpinx.

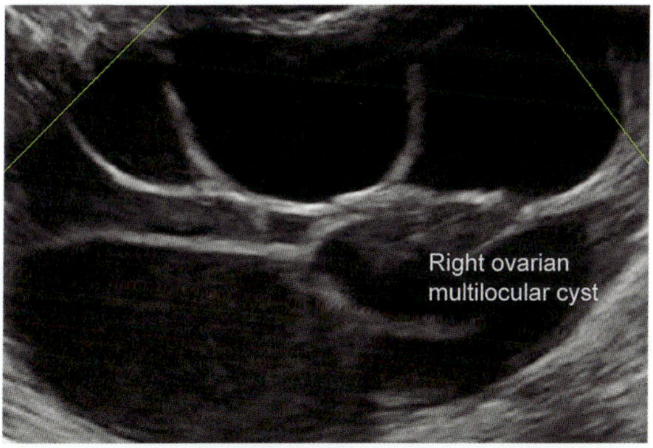

Fig. 8: Multilocular cyst.

- Typical peritoneal inclusion cyst (any size)
- *Typical hydrosalpinx (any size):* Incomplete septations, endosalpingeal folds **(Fig. 7)**

  Management: Typically, these masses do not require further intervention unless they are symptomatic or increase in size. Follow-up imaging may be considered based on patient age, symptoms, or size of the mass.

4. *O-RADS3—Low risk of malignancy:* Masses in this category have a 1–<10% risk of malignancy. Examples include:
   - *Unilocular cysts (≥10 cm) with one thin septation:* The cyst contains a single thin septation (<3 mm) but no solid components.
   - *Typical dermoid/hemorrhagic cyst/endometrioma cysts (≥10 cm)*
   - Multilocular cyst with smooth inner wall (<10 cm), color score 1–3 (No to moderate flow) **(Fig. 8)**
   - Solid/solid appearing (≥80%) with smooth contour, any size, color score 1 (No flow)

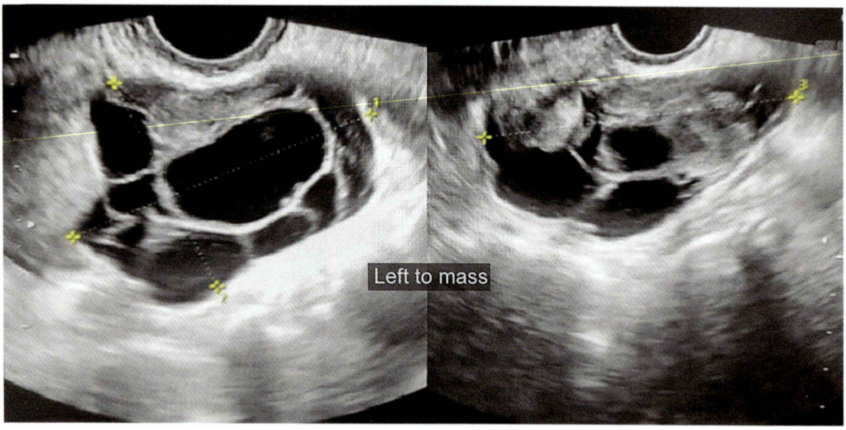

Fig. 9: Multilocular cysts.

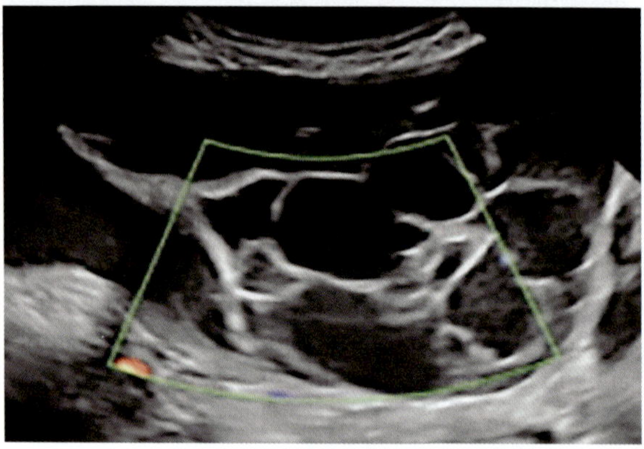

Fig. 10: Multilocular cysts.

Management: Follow-up ultrasound is recommended for 6-12 months to monitor for changes in size or characteristics. Referral to a gynecologist is advised if the mass persists or grows.

5. *O-RADS4—Intermediate risk of malignancy:* Masses in this category have a 10–<50% risk of malignancy and may display features such as:
   - Multilocular cysts with smooth inner wall (≥10 cm), color score 1–3 **(Fig. 9)**
   - Multilocular cysts with smooth inner wall (any size), color score 4 (very strong flow)
   - Multilocular cysts with irregular inner wall and/or irregular septation, any size, any color score **(Fig. 10)**
   - Multilocular cyst with solid/solid appearing component, no papillary projections, any size, color score 1–2 (No to mild flow)

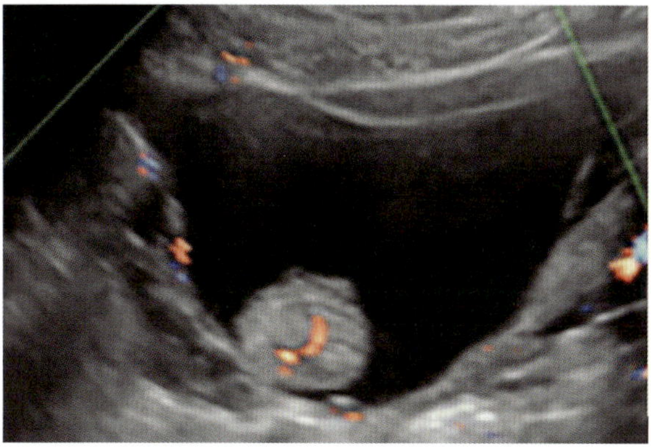

Fig. 11: Unilocular cyst.

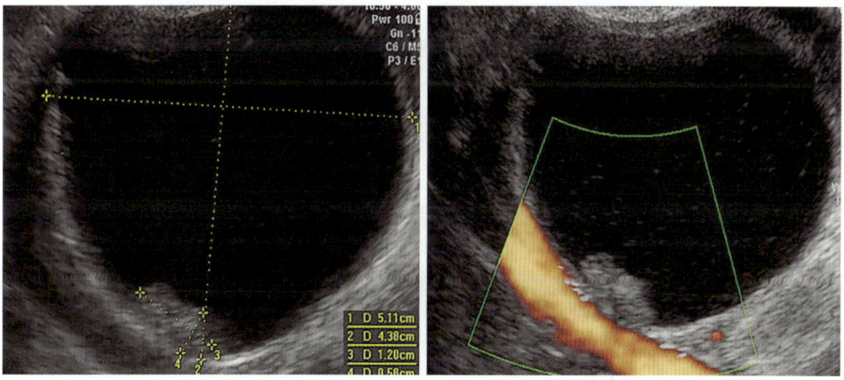

Fig. 12: Unilocular cysts.

- Unilocular cyst with solid/solid appearing components, no papillary projections, any size, any color score **(Fig. 11)**
- *Unilocular cysts with 1–3 papillary projections, any size, any color score* **(Fig. 12)**
- Solid (≥80%) with smooth contour, any size, color score 2–3 (mild-to-moderate flow) **(Fig. 13)**

  Management: Referral to a gynecologic oncologist is recommended for further evaluation and possible surgical intervention.

6. *O-RADS5—High Risk of malignancy:* Masses in this category have a ≥50% risk of malignancy. These are characterized by:
   - Unilocular cysts with ≥4 papillary projections, any size, any color score
   - Multilocular cyst with solid component, any size, color score 4 (moderate to very strong flow) **(Fig. 14)**

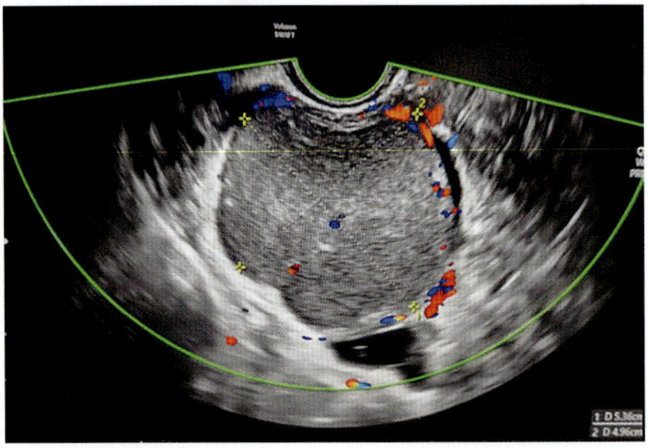

Fig. 13: Solid (≥80%) with smooth contour.

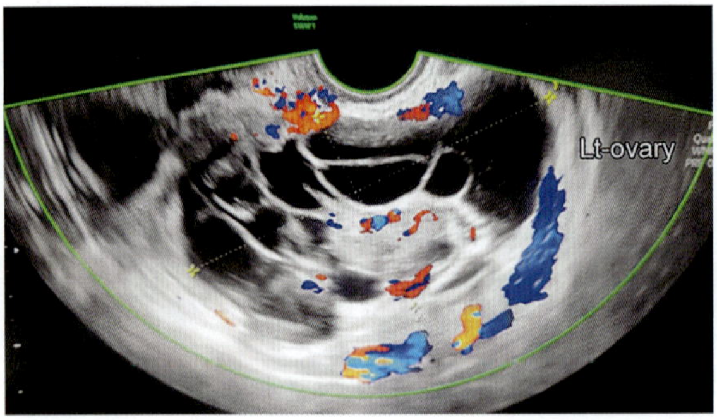

Fig. 14: Multilocular cyst.

- Solid (≥80%) with smooth contour, any size, color score 4
- Solid/solid appearing (≥80%) with irregular contour, any size, any color score
- Ascites and/or peritoneal nodules

  Management: Urgent referral to a gynecologic oncologist is warranted for timely surgical evaluation and appropriate management.

CONCLUSION

O-RADS is a valuable tool in the ultrasonographic assessment of adnexal masses, providing a standardized approach to risk stratification and management. By utilizing this system, clinicians can more effectively determine the likelihood of malignancy, ensure appropriate follow-up, and optimize patient outcomes. Regular use of O-RADS in clinical practice can enhance diagnostic accuracy, streamline communication, and ultimately improve patient care.

REFERENCES

1. RCOG/BSGE Joint Guideline I November 2011.
2. Green-top Guideline No. 34 July 2016, RCOG.
3. Smorgick N, Maymon R. Assessment of adnexal masses using ultrasound: a practical review. Int J Womens Health. 2014;6:857-63. Published online 2014 Sep 23. doi: 10.2147/IJWH.S47075.
4. Carvalho JP, Moretti-Marques R, Filho ALDS. Adnexal mass: diagnosis and management. Rev Bras Ginecol Obstet. 2020;42(7):438-43. doi: 10.1055/s-0040-1715547.
5. Lee SJ, Oh HR, Na S, Hwang HS, Lee SM. Ultrasonographic ovarian mass scoring system for predicting malignancy in pregnant women with ovarian mass. Obstet Gynecol Sci. 2022;65(1):1–13. Published online 2022 Jan 15. doi: 10.5468/ogs.21212.
6. Garg S, Kaur A, Mohi JK, Sibia PK, Kaur N. Evaluation of IOTA simple ultrasound rules to distinguish benign and malignant ovarian tumours. J Clin Diagn Res. 2017;11(8):TC06–TC09. Published online 2017 Aug 1. doi: 10.7860/JCDR/2017/26790.10353.
7. O-RADS US Risk Stratification and Management System, https://doi.org/10.1148/radiol.2019191150.

3

CHAPTER

First-Trimester Anomalies

Chanchal Singh, Vrunda Appannagari

INTRODUCTION

Fetal structural malformations are seen in 2–4% of all pregnancies. It is estimated that 1.7 million birth defects occur annually and constitute a leading cause of stillbirth and neonatal deaths. In most countries including ours, targeted imaging for fetal anomaly is usually performed at 18–22 weeks of gestation. The first-trimester scan is primarily used for dating, assessing viability, detecting multiple pregnancies, and evaluating markers for Down syndrome. In the last few decades, a better understanding of fetal development, availability of high-resolution ultrasound machines, increasing expertise in fetal medicine and wide application of the nuchal translucency (NT) scan, first-trimester USG has essentially preponed the anomaly scan from the mid-trimester to the first trimester. The advent of noninvasive prenatal screening (NIPS), which has a much higher sensitivity and specificity for detection of Down syndrome as compared to the combined first-trimester screening, has also shifted the focus of first-trimester ultrasound to early detection of structural abnormalities.

FIRST-TRIMESTER ULTRASOUND

The first-trimester ultrasound is performed at 11 weeks to 13 weeks and 6 days, corresponding to a crown to rump length (CRL) of 45–84 mm. It includes assessment of viability, multiple pregnancy and chorionicity, measurement of CRL, nuchal translucency (NT), assessment of nasal bone (NB), ductus venosus and tricuspid regurgitation as part of screening for Down syndrome. Uterine artery Dopplers are done for risk assessment for preeclampsia. The new ISUOG guideline issued in 2023 also recommends assessment of the complete fetal structure in addition to screening for trisomy 21 and preeclampsia. Both transabdominal and transvaginal ultrasound can be used to assess the fetus. With obesity becoming a global epidemic, use of transvaginal ultrasound in the first trimester is a golden opportunity for early detection of structural abnormalities in women with high BMI.

Table 1 enlists the fetal structures and the views that should be obtained at the first-trimester ultrasound. **Figure 1** shows the ultrasound images that should be obtained in the first trimester.

Detection rates of 30–60% for all major structural anomalies have been reported with an extremely low false-positive rate (0.04%).[1,2] Amongst the first such studies, Syngelaki et al. categorized first-trimester abnormalities as 'always detectable,' 'potentially detectable,' and 'undetectable.'[1]

Factors affecting detection rates of structural abnormalities in the first trimester include following a standardized protocol, use of transvaginal ultrasound, operator experience, use of standardized equipment, maternal characteristics like body mass index (BMI) and multiple pregnancy.[3] Syngelaki et al. emphasize that recognizing an additional 42% of potentially detectable anomalies depending on these factors.[1] The use of a standardized protocol is reported to be associated with a 2-fold increased detection rate.[4]

Table 2 enlists the categorization of abnormalities that can be detected in the first trimester.

TABLE 1: Checklist for first trimester early morphology scan.

Fetal head	• Cranial bones • Midline Falx • Choroid plexus filling the ventricles (butterfly sign)
Mid sagittal view of fetal face and neck	• Normal profile • Nasal bone ('equal to' sign) • Nuchal translucency • Rectangular palate (vomer and palatine bone) • Intracranial translucency
Axial view of fetal face	• Eyes with lens • Retronasal triangle • Normal mandible (mandibular gap)
Thorax	• Symmetrical lungs • No effusion • Situs • Fetal heart rate • Cardiac axis • 4 symmetrical chambers of heart • 3 vessel view
Abdomen	• Stomach bubble • Cord insertion and three vessel cord • Bladder • Kidneys
Extremities	• All three segments of all four limbs • Hand and feet with normal orientation and movements
Spine	Vertebrae with intact overlying skin
Placenta	Size, texture, placental cord insertion

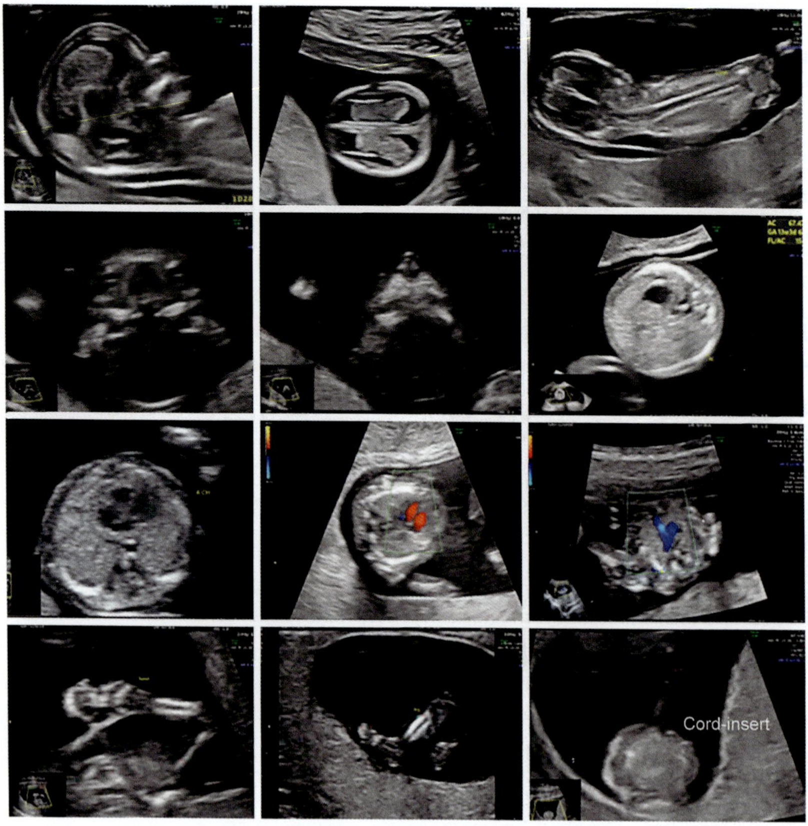

Fig. 1: Images that should be obtained at the first-trimester ultrasound.

TABLE 2: Abnormalities detectable in the first trimester.

Always detectable	*Potentially detectable*	*Not detectable*
Acrania	Micrognathia	Agenesis of corpus callosum
Exencephaly	Cleft lip and palate	Bladder exstrophy
Holoprosencephaly	Anophthalmia, microphthalmia	Congenital pulmonary adenomatoid malformation (CPAM)
Gastroschisis, exomphalos	Sacral agenesis	Extralobar pulmonary sequestration
Megacystis	Sacrococcygeal teratoma*	Clubfoot
Body stalk anomaly	Diaphragmatic hernia*	Duodenal atresia
Limb reduction defects	Hypoplastic left/right heart	Bowel obstruction
Univentricular heart	Transposition of great arteries	Hydronephrosis, Duplex kidneys
Conjoined twins	Tetralogy of Fallot	CNS cortical abnormalities
Sirenomelia	Arthrogryposis	Cerebellar hypoplasia

*If large enough to be seen at this gestation.

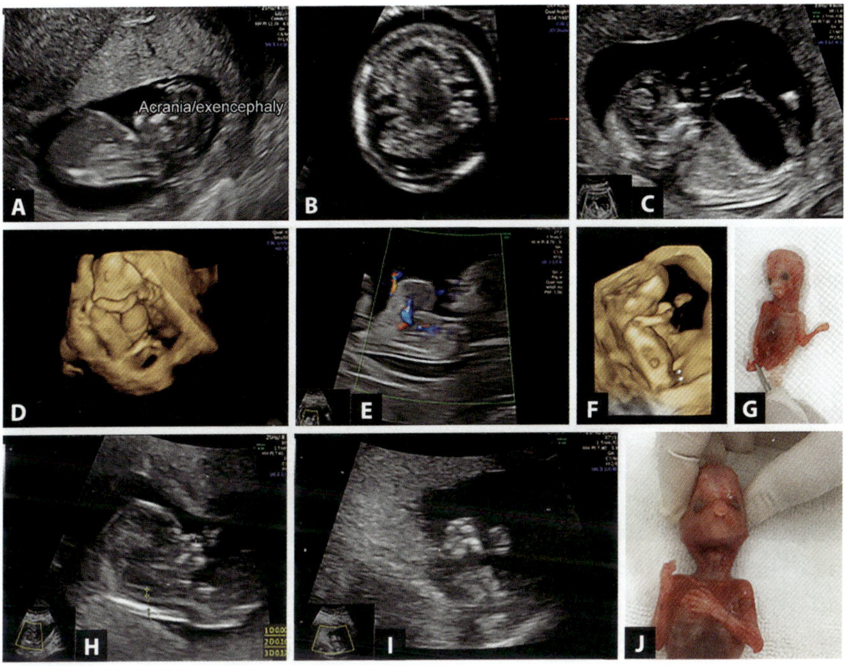

Figs. 2A to J: Potentially detectable abnormalities in first trimester. (A) Acrania/exencephaly; (B) Holoprosencephaly; (C) Megacystis; (D and E) Exomphalos; (F and G) Caudal regression syndrome; (H to J) Bilateral cleft lip and palate.

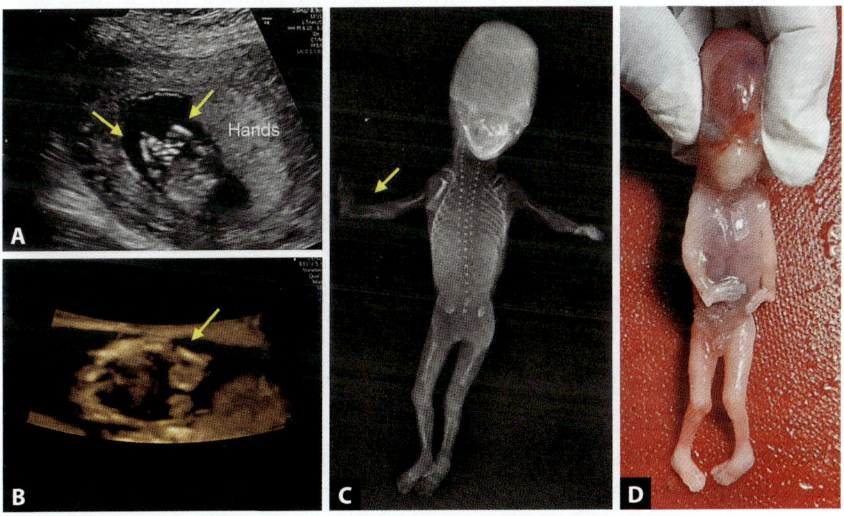

Figs. 3A to D: Bilateral radial aplasia detected in the first trimester.

Figures 2 to 4 provide examples of detectable abnormalities in the first trimester.

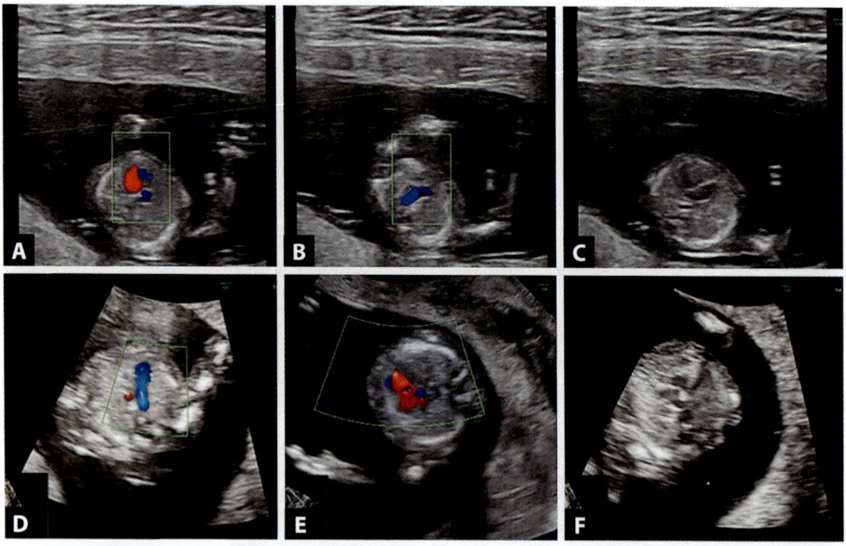

Figs. 4A to F: Hypoplastic left heart (A to C); Hypoplastic right heart (D to F)

ADVANTAGES OF EARLY DETECTION OF ABNORMALITIES

An early diagnosis of fetal abnormality can help clinicians and parents make decisions by allowing sufficient time for additional investigations, i.e., diagnostic testing for fetal aneuploidy and further genetic testing like microarray and/or whole exome sequencing which have a turn-around time of 2–4 weeks. The detection of a structural abnormality can also help choose diagnostic testing over cfDNA as the next test, thereby avoiding unnecessary delays in diagnosis and optimizing resources. The time available for test results and post-test counseling becomes critical due to legal limits for the termination. Early diagnosis of correctable abnormalities allows early involvement of a multidisciplinary team and will help in optimizing both maternal and neonatal outcomes.

LIMITATIONS OF FIRST-TRIMESTER EARLY MORPHOLOGY SCAN

Although very low false positive rates are reported for the 'always detectable' abnormalities in the first trimester,[5] it is prudent to advise a follow-up scan after 2–4 weeks for some abnormalities especially cardiac anomalies. The first-trimester early morphology scan does not replace a detailed second-trimester targeted scan for fetal anomalies. Many anomalies suspected in the first trimester may need confirmation for definitive diagnosis in the second trimester. It is extremely important for centers to audit their practice and to ensure confirmation of the abnormalities detected at the first trimester either after birth or by autopsy if termination is opted for.

CONCLUSION

First-trimester ultrasound using the standard protocol can effectively identify a large proportion of the "potentially detectable" in the first trimester, apart from always detectable ones. It is especially useful in women with high BMI as the transvaginal route provides better imaging quality than a mid-trimester scan. However, it is essential to emphasize that all defects cannot be detected in the first trimester due to the late manifestation, and subsequent ultrasound for detailed anomaly screening in the mid-trimester is recommended.

REFERENCES

1. Syngelaki A, Hammami A, Bower S, Zidere V, Akolekar R, Nicolaides KH. Diagnosis of fetal non-chromosomal abnormalities on routine ultrasound examination at 11–13 weeks' gestation. Ultrasound Obstet Gynecol. 2019;54(4):468-76.
2. Singh C, Shahnaz G, Dagar S, Shastri A, Kurana D, Thakur S. Performance of first-trimester ultrasound in detection of structural abnormalities in Indian women: a prospective observational study. Int J Gynecol Obstet. 2023;160(3):1042-3.
3. Karim JN, Roberts NW, Salomon LJ, Papageorghiou AT. Systematic review of first-trimester ultrasound screening for detection of fetal structural anomalies and factors that affect screening performance. Ultrasound Obstet Gynecol. 2017;50(4):429-41.
4. Liao Y, Wen H, Ouyang S, et al. Routine first-trimester ultrasound screening using a standardized anatomical protocol. Am J Obstet Gynecol. 2021;224(4):396.e1-e15.
5. Buijtendijk MF, Bet BB, Leeflang MM, Shah H, Reuvekamp T, Goring T, et al. Diagnostic accuracy of ultrasound screening for fetal structural abnormalities during the first and second trimester of pregnancy in low-risk and unselected populations. Cochrane Database Syst Rev. 2024;5(5):CD014715.

4 CHAPTER

Basics of Obstetric Doppler: A Comprehensive Overview

Prasanna Roy

INTRODUCTION

Obstetric Doppler ultrasound plays a pivotal role in evaluating fetal health, particularly in high-risk pregnancies. This non-invasive tool is essential in assessing fetal circulation and placental function, guiding clinical management to prevent adverse perinatal outcomes. Doppler ultrasound offers invaluable information for monitoring fetal well-being, especially in cases of fetal growth restriction (FGR), pre-eclampsia, and other placental pathologies.[1-3]

DOPPLER PHYSICS

The Doppler effect, first described by Christian Doppler, is the change in frequency of a wave as the source and observer move relative to each other. The frequency shift between the transmitted and received sound waves allows for the calculation of the velocity of blood flow.[4-6] *Accurate Doppler measurements depend on the angle of insonation. Ideally, this should be as close to 0° as possible for accurate velocity measurement. For practical reasons, an angle of less than 30° is recommended, as higher angles increase measurement errors.*

Pulsed-wave Doppler

This technique allows for the precise localization of blood flow by adjusting the sample volume to a specific region of interest. It is most commonly used in obstetric imaging because of its ability to selectively sample blood flow from specific fetal vessels **(Figs. 1 and 2)**.

Continuous-wave Doppler

While it can detect higher velocities, continuous-wave Doppler lacks spatial resolution and is rarely used in fetal assessment.

Color Doppler and Power Doppler

These techniques map blood flow direction and velocity across an area, with color Doppler used to assess the direction of blood flow and power Doppler

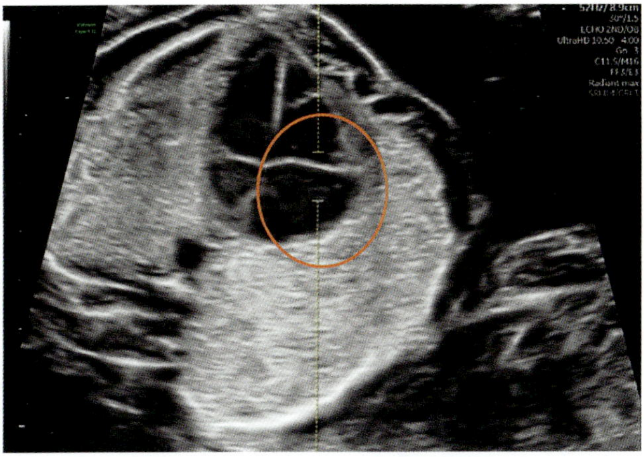

Fig. 1: Placement of Doppler gate.

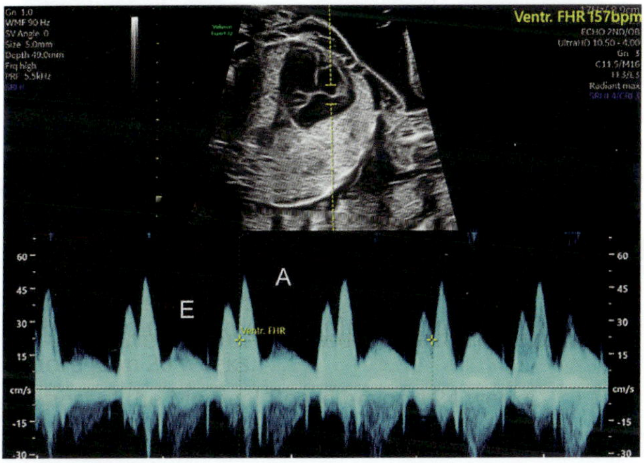

Fig. 2: *Spectral Doppler waveform:* Normally, the A wave is usually greater, although as gestation progresses, the E/A ratio increases. Normally E/A ratio is <1.

being more sensitive to low-flow velocities, such as those seen in small fetal vessels **(Figs. 3 and 4)**.

KEY DOPPLER PARAMETERS

Pulsatility index (PI): PI is a measure of blood flow pulsatility. It reflects downstream resistance, and higher values suggest increased resistance to flow.

Resistance index (RI): RI is another indicator of vascular resistance.

Systolic/Diastolic (S/D) ratio: This ratio compares the systolic and diastolic velocities in the vessel of interest. An increasing S/D ratio often reflects placental insufficiency.

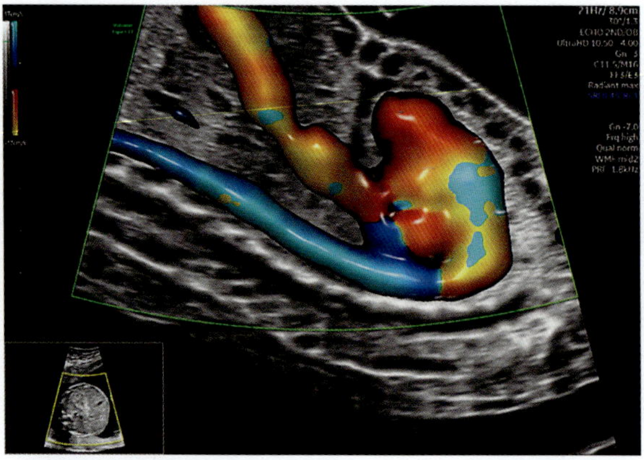

Fig. 3: Color Doppler.

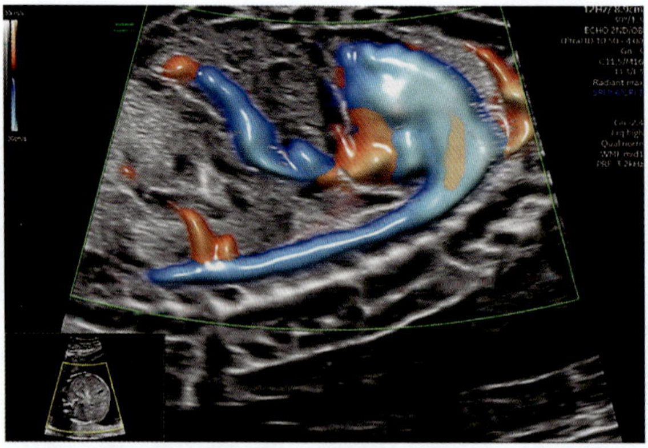

Fig. 4: Power Doppler.

IMAGE ACQUISITION

- *Angle of insonation:* Ideally, the angle between the ultrasound beam and the direction of blood flow should be ≤30° to avoid significant errors in velocity measurement.
- *Sample volume:* Should be placed at the center of the vessel and adjusted to cover the entire lumen.

INDICATIONS FOR OBSTETRIC DOPPLER

Fetal growth restriction (FGR): To assess placental insufficiency and fetal well-being.

Pre-eclampsia: Early prediction and monitoring of this hypertensive disorder, often associated with poor placental perfusion.

Multiple pregnancies: Especially in cases of sIUGR, TTTS, and TRAP complications in monochorionic twins.

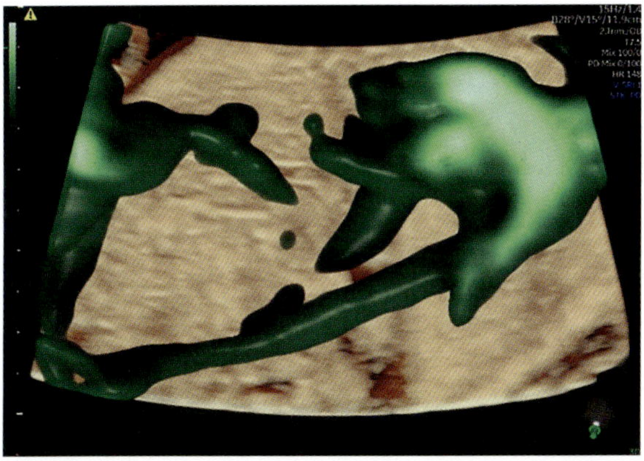

Fig. 5: Example of congenital anomalies where Doppler is used—DV agenesis.

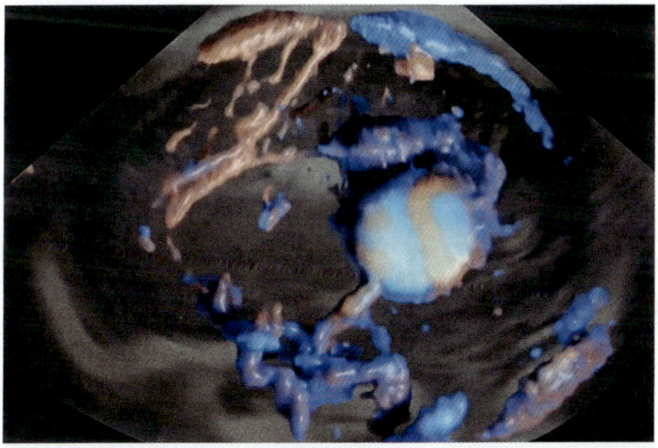

Fig. 6: Example of congenital anomalies where Doppler is used—Vein of Galen aneurysm.

Fetal echocardiography and fetal anemia.

Diagnosis of congenital anomalies involving the vascular system, e.g., vein of Galen aneurysm **(Figs. 5 and 6)**.

Maternal conditions: Placenta accreta spectrum and medical disorders such as diabetes, lupus, and chronic hypertension, where placental function may be compromised.

KEY VESSELS ASSESSED IN OBSTETRIC DOPPLER[7-9]

Umbilical Artery Doppler

Umbilical artery Doppler provides information about placental resistance and placental function. It is the primary modality for assessing placental insufficiency in fetal growth restriction (FGR) **(Fig. 7)**.

Increased PI/RI indicates increased placental resistance.

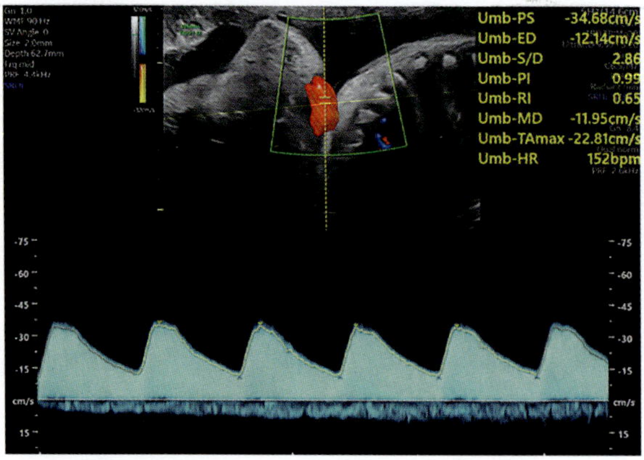

Fig. 7: Normal umbilical artery Doppler.

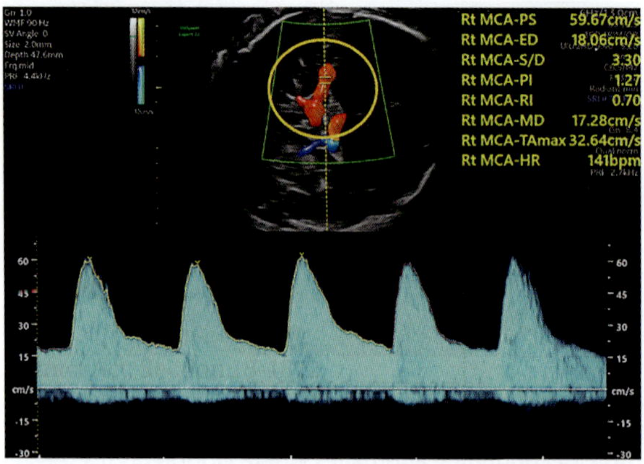

Fig. 8: Normal MCA Doppler waveform (note the 0° angle of insonation).

Absent or reversed end-diastolic flow (AREDF) signifies critical placental insufficiency, requiring urgent intervention.

Middle Cerebral Artery Doppler

- Middle cerebral artery (MCA) Doppler evaluates the cerebral blood flow in the fetus and is primarily used to assess fetal hypoxia and anemia **(Fig. 8)**.
- *A decreased PI suggests a brain-sparing effect, indicating fetal hypoxia.*
- *Elevated PSV is predictive of fetal anemia, particularly in cases of isoimmunization or parvovirus infection (MCA-PSV Mom >1.5).*
- It can sometimes show end diastolic flow reversal, which is generally due to increased intracranial pressure, mostly by probe compression (non-pathological finding) **(Fig. 8)**.

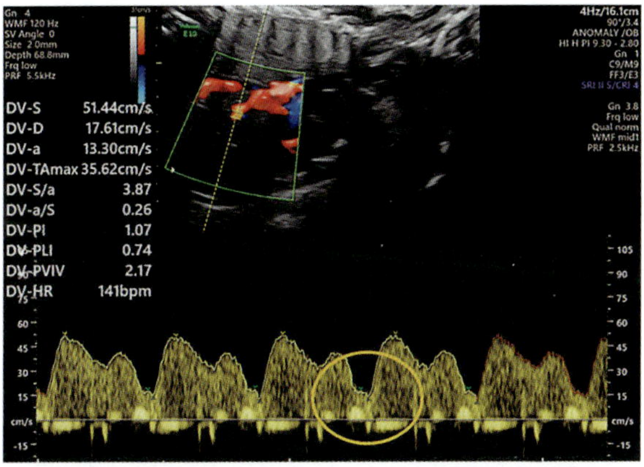

Fig. 9: Normal DV Doppler with positive A-wave.

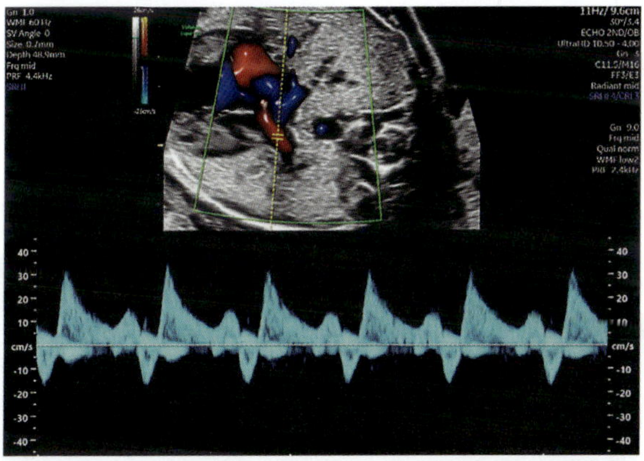

Fig. 10: Reversal of A-wave in DV Doppler.

Ductus Venosus Doppler

- Ductus venosus (DV) Doppler is valuable in evaluating fetal cardiac function, especially in the context of FGR or fetal hydrops. It reflects the cardiac preload and venous return to the heart.
- A reversed or absent A-wave suggests right ventricular dysfunction and is often associated with aneuploidy and poor perinatal outcomes.
- DV PI up to 1.3—negative marker for trisomy 21
- DV PI >1.3—positive marker for trisomy 21 **(Figs. 9 and 10)**

Uterine Artery Doppler

Uterine artery Doppler assesses the blood flow to the placenta from the maternal side and is used to predict pre-eclampsia and FGR.

Increased PI/RI or the presence of notching in the second trimester is predictive of placental insufficiency and a higher risk of pre-eclampsia or FGR **(Figs. 11 and 12)**.

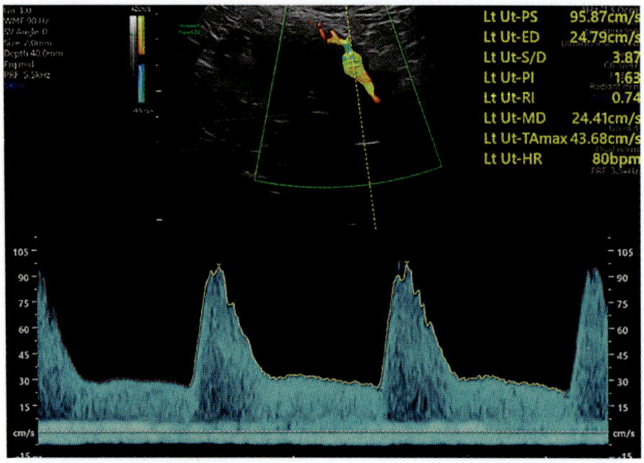

Fig. 11: Normal uterine artery Doppler waveform.

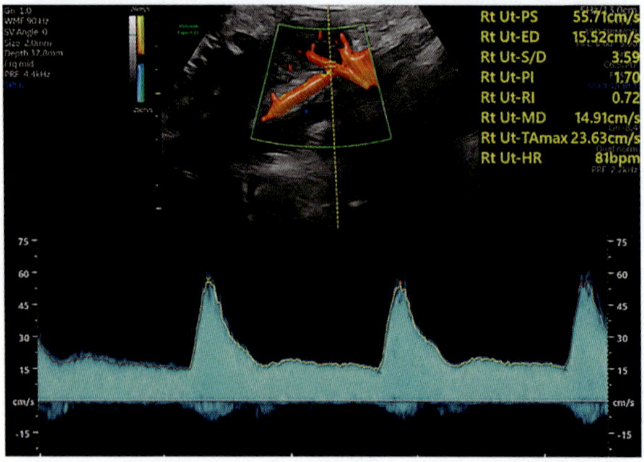

Fig. 12: High-resistance uterine artery Doppler with notching (high PI).

CLINICAL APPLICATIONS OF OBSTETRIC DOPPLER ULTRASOUND

Uterine Artery Doppler

The Doppler assessment is conducted at 11–13+6 weeks and again at 20–24 weeks of gestation. The transducer is placed on the lower abdomen, and the uterine arteries are identified at the level of the internal os. *The mean PI of right and left sides is measured, and should be >95th centile.*

Interpretation: Ut PI reduced by 0.75 each trimester.

In 1st trimester >2.5, 2nd trimester >1.75, and 3rd trimester >1.

Umbilical Artery Doppler

The umbilical artery is assessed by placing the transducer on the maternal abdomen and visualizing the umbilical cord. The Doppler sample volume

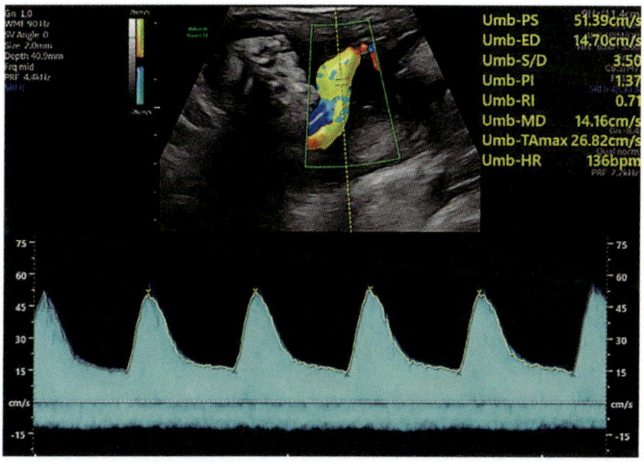

Fig. 13: Pulsatile umbilical Doppler (High PI at 35 weeks).

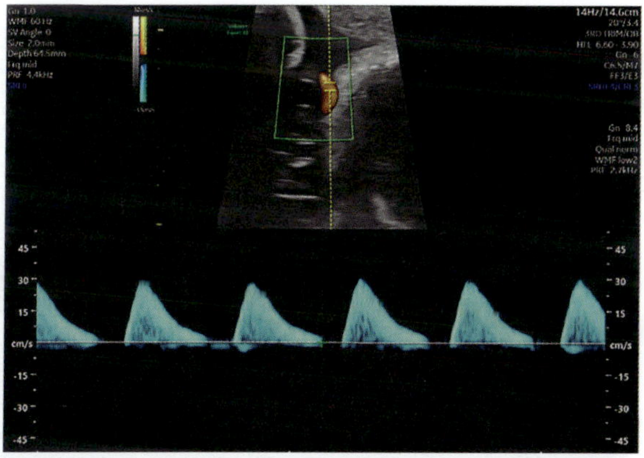

Fig. 14: Absent end diastolic flow (AEDF) in umbilical Doppler.

is placed in a free-floating loop of the cord, and the PI is measured **(Figs. 13 to 15)**.

Interpretation:

- *Normal findings:* Continuous forward flow throughout the cardiac cycle, with a normal PI for gestational age.
- *Abnormal findings:* Absent or reversed end-diastolic flow, indicating severe placental insufficiency and increased risk of perinatal morbidity and mortality.

Middle Cerebral Artery Doppler

The MCA is visualized in a transverse section of the fetal head at the level of the sphenoid bones. The Doppler sample volume is placed in the proximal third of the MCA, and the peak systolic velocity (PSV) is measured **(Figs. 16 to 18)**.

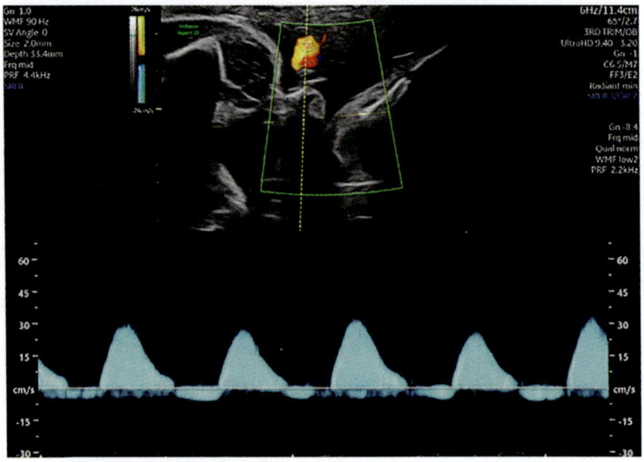

Fig. 15: Reversal of end diastolic flow (REDF).

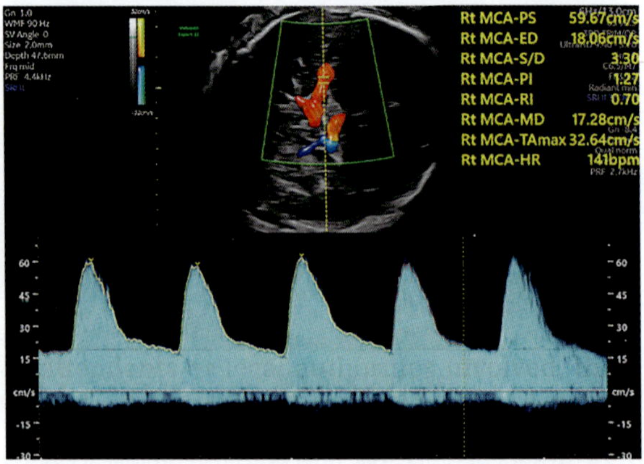

Fig. 16: Decreased PI of MCA Doppler in fetal hypoxia.

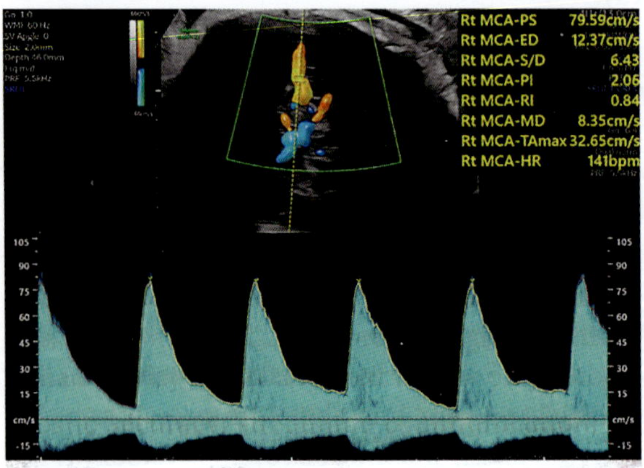

Fig. 17: Increased PSV of MCA Doppler in fetal anemia.

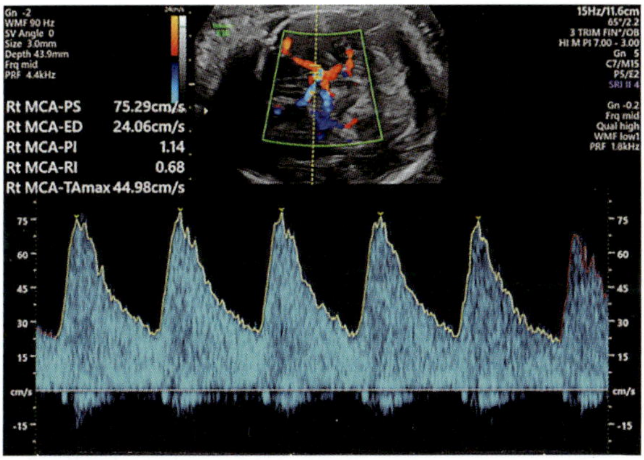

Fig. 18: Paradoxical MCA. In cases of severe hypoxia, when the vasodilatation ability is exhausted, the flow can revert back to a high resistance pattern, which is a very poor prognostic sign.

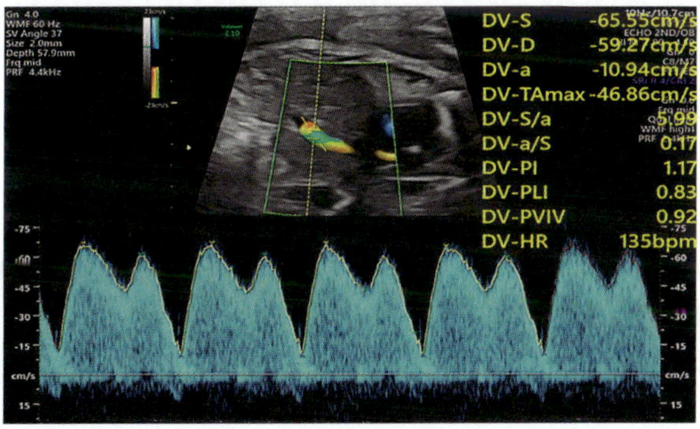

Fig. 19: Pulsatile DV Doppler in eFGR.

Interpretation:
- *Normal findings:* PI within the normal range for gestational age.
- *Abnormal findings:* Decreased PI or increased PSV, suggesting fetal hypoxia or anemia. An increased PSV is a sensitive marker for fetal anemia.

Ductus Venosus Doppler[10]

The ductus venosus is visualized in a sagittal section of the fetal abdomen. The Doppler sample volume is placed at the inlet of the ductus venosus with a gate of 0.7–1 mm, and the waveform is assessed for the presence of the A-wave **(Fig. 19)**.

Interpretation:
- *Normal findings:* Positive A-wave, indicating normal cardiac function.
- *Abnormal findings:* Reversed A-wave, indicating cardiac compromise and poor prognosis. This finding is associated with increased perinatal morbidity and mortality.

Cerebroplacental Ratio (CPR)

Indications: The cerebroplacental ratio (CPR) is used to assess the balance between fetal cerebral and placental blood flow. It is particularly useful in the management of IUGR.

Technique: The CPR is calculated by dividing the PI of the MCA by the PI of the umbilical artery.

CPR is below 5th centile if: CPR is 1.2 between 30-35 weeks OR CPR is 1.0 after 35 weeks.

Interpretation ***(Table 1)****:*

- *Normal CPR:* Indicates balanced blood flow between the brain and placenta.
- *Low CPR:* Suggests brain-sparing, a compensatory mechanism due to placental insufficiency, and is associated with adverse perinatal outcomes.

CLASSIFICATION OF FGR BASED ON DELPHI CONSENSUS

Management of FGR based on Doppler Findings (Table 2)

Stages of FGR based on Doppler findings are described in **Table 2**.

TABLE 1: Doppler in fetal growth restriction (FGR).

• *Early FGR (GA <32 weeks):* Absence of congenital anomalies • EFW or AC <3rd percentile OR UA-AEDF Or • EFW/AC <10th centile combined with: – UtA PI >95th centile – UA PI >95th centile	• *Late FGR (GA ≥32 weeks):* Absence of congenital anomalies • *EFW/AC <3rd centile:* Or 2 out of 3: • EFW/AC <10th centile EFW/AC crossing centiles >2 quartiles on growth centiles • CPR <5th centile or UA-PI >95th centile

TABLE 2: Stages of FGR based on Doppler findings.

Stage	*Pathophysiological correlate*	*Criteria (any of)*	*Monitoring*	*GA/Mode of delivery*
1	Severe smallness or mild placental insufficiency	• EFW <3rd centile • CPR <p5 • UA-PI >p95 • MCA-PI <p5 • Ut-PI >p95	Weekly	37 weeks LI
2	Severe placental insufficiency	• UA-AEDV • Reverse AoI	Biweekly	34 weeks CS
3	Low suspicion fetal acidosis	• UA-REDV • DV-PI >p95	1–2 days	30 weeks CS
4	High suspicion fetal acidosis	• DV reverse a flow • cCTG <3 ms • FHR decelerations	12 hourly	26 weeks CS

DOPPLER IN TWIN-TWIN TRANSFUSION SYNDROME (TTTS)

TTTS is a serious complication in monochorionic twin pregnancies, where abnormal placental vascular connections cause an imbalance in blood flow between the twins. Doppler ultrasound plays a vital role in diagnosing and monitoring TTTS **(Table 3)**.

Doppler of the donor twin typically shows increased resistance in the umbilical artery and MCA Doppler, while the recipient twin often exhibits reversed or absent end-diastolic flow in the umbilical artery and abnormal ductus venosus flow **(Fig. 20)**.

At 11–14 weeks scan, chance of developing TTTS triples if one of the DV flow is abnormal.

TABLE 3: Stages of twin-twin transfusion syndrome (TTTS) (Quintero staging).

Stage I	Donor bladder visible
Stage II	• No donor bladder • Normal Doppler assessments
Stage III	• Abnormal Doppler assessments • *For donor:* – AEDF/REDF in donor umbilical artery +/– • *For recipient:* – Abnormal DV flow – Pulsatile umbilical vein
Stage IV	Hydrops in one twin
Stage V	Death of one/both twins

Doppler in selective FGR

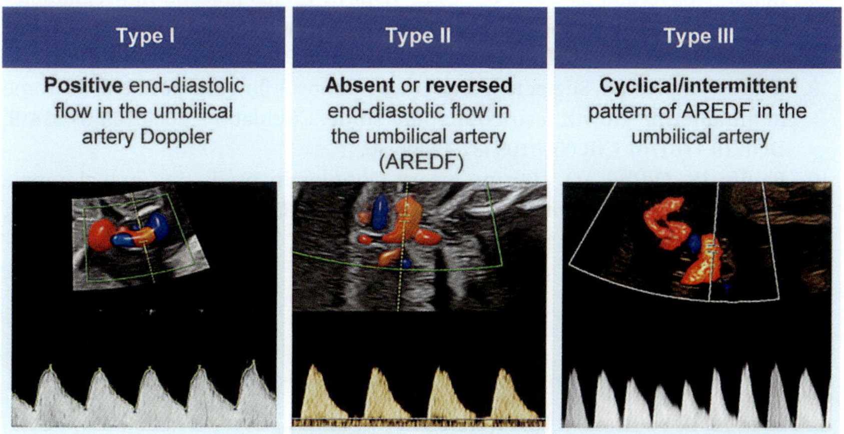

Fig. 20: Doppler in selective FGR in twins.

CONCLUSION

Obstetric Doppler ultrasound is a powerful tool in the assessment of fetal and placental circulation. It provides critical insights into fetal well-being, particularly in high-risk pregnancies such as those affected by fetal growth restriction, pre-eclampsia, and twin-twin transfusion syndrome. Guidelines from ISUOG, ACOG, SMFM, and the RCOG consistently recommend the use of Doppler as an essential part of the surveillance in these pregnancies, with umbilical artery, MCA, and ductus venosus Doppler being the most frequently utilized studies.

REFERENCES

1. ISUOG Practice Guidelines: use of Doppler ultrasonography in obstetrics. Ultrasound Obstet Gynecol. 2013;41:233-9.
2. ACOG Practice Bulletin No. 134: Fetal Growth Restriction. Obstet Gynecol. 2013;121:1122-33.
3. SMFM Consult Series #41: Doppler assessment of the fetus with intrauterine growth restriction. Am J Obstet Gynecol. 2018;218:B2-8.
4. RCOG Green-top Guideline No. 31: The Investigation and Management of the Small-for-Gestational-Age Fetus, 2014.
5. Alfirevic Z, Stampalija T, Gyte GM. Fetal and umbilical Doppler ultrasound in high-risk pregnancies. Cochrane Database of Systematic Reviews. 2015(2) DOI: 10.1002/14651858.CD007529.pub4.
6. Oepkes D, Seaward G, Vandenbussche F, et al. Middle cerebral artery Doppler ultrasonography to predict fetal anemia before invasive testing in red-cell alloimmunization. New England Journal of Medicine. 2006;355(2):156-64. DOI: 10.1056/NEJMoa052706.
7. Lees C, Marlow N, Arabin B, et al. Perinatal morbidity and mortality in early-onset fetal growth restriction: cohort outcomes of the trial of randomized umbilical and fetal flow in Europe (TRUFFLE). Ultrasound Obstet Gynecol. 2013;42(4):400-08. DOI: 10.1002/uog.13190.
8. Rolnik DL, Wright D, Poon LC, et al. Aspirin versus placebo in pregnancies at high risk for preterm preeclampsia. New England Journal of Medicine. 2017;377(7):613-22. DOI: 10.1056/NEJMoa1704559.
9. Bilardo CM, Wolf H, Stigter RH, et al. Ductus venosus flow and perinatal outcome in intrauterine growth restriction: pilot study. Circulation. 2004;109(3):114-9. DOI: 10.1161/01.CIR.0000109487.49306.36.
10. Bamfo JE, Odibo AO. Uterine artery Doppler in predicting preeclampsia and intrauterine growth restriction. Reviews in Obstetrics and Gynecology. 2011;4(1):28-37. PMID: 22102928.

5

CHAPTER

Late Onset Anomalies

Debasmita Mandal

BACKGROUND

The primary objective of obstetric ultrasonography is the prenatal detection of congenital anomalies. Over the past 30 years, significant advancements have been made in diagnosing even minor or subtle fetal anomalies. These improvements are largely due to enhanced equipment, greater examiner experience, and more comprehensive training. Despite these advances, a considerable number of fetal anomalies remain undiagnosed, even by highly skilled and experienced sonographers using state-of-the-art technology. These diagnostic failures are often attributed to misinterpretations or errors in diagnosis.

So, it is important to realize though inadvertent mistakes happen there are some factors which play a crucial role in this mishappening.

1. The fetal embryological developmental ladder has its own course of events though out the pregnancy.
2. Few organs are developed early structurally but functionally represent later especially fetal heart.
3. Few other organs develop structurally and functionally throughout the gestation, especially the fetal brain.
4. Though all parameters are in normal pace during all fetal scans, but growth of fetal long bones may arrest just some weeks before last trimester.
5. Intrauterine growth retardation may happen after 32 weeks as well.
6. Even fetal disease pathologies progress with advancement of pregnancy, to be detected and prognosticated in better way during later gestation.

So, it is very important to analyze the issue of late anomalies rather to blame on logistic problems.

TYPES

A nice classification for categorizing the pathologies involved in evolving anomalies has been put forth by Dr Simcha Yagel and Dr Reuwen Achiron.[1] (**Flowchart 1 and Table 1**)

Flowchart 1: Classification for categorizing the pathologies involved in evolving anomalies.

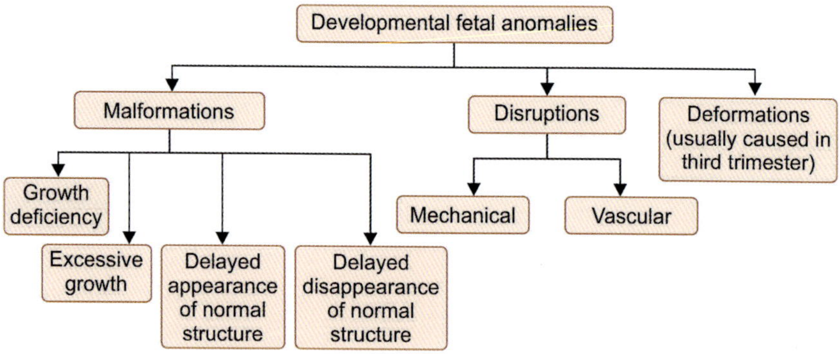

Source: Yagel S, Achiron R. Developmental fetal malformations: time to change the terminology. Ultrasound Obstet Gynaecol. 1998;11:89-91.

TABLE 1: List of structural anomalies with possible intrauterine evolvement.

Malformations	***Disruptions***
Growth deficiency: • X-linked hydrocephalous • Duodenal atresia • Urinary tract dilation/Hydronephrosis • Achondroplasia • Great vessel stenosis • Premature closure foramen of ovale • Bowel atresia • Anal atresia	*Mechanical:* Amniotic band syndrome
Excessive growth: • Chorioangioma • Sacrococcygeal teratoma • Neuroblastoma • Rhabdomyoma • Remodeling of heart in GDM, IUGR, TTTS • Cardiomyopathy • Ventricular aneurysm	*Vascular:* • Terminal limb reduction • Intrauterine coronary occlusion
Delayed appearance of normal structure: • Dandy–Walker malformation • Agenesis of corpus callosum • Vein of Galen malformation • Cortical migration disorders	*Infections:* Hemorrhage
Delayed disappearance of normal structure: • Choroid plexus cysts • Abdominal cyst • Cervical blebs • Patent ductus arteriosus	

Many fetal anomalies develop during pregnancy, though there is limited data on their progression. Several cases from various studies are recapitulated in **Table 1**.

For example, in X-linked hydrocephalus, the underdevelopment of the aqueduct of Silvius becomes noticeable only after the 16th week of gestation.

In duodenal atresia, the underlying issue, caused by a failure in the recanalization of the duodenum, occurs around 7–8 weeks of gestation, but its effects are only visible by mid-trimester **(Fig. 1)**.

Abdominal cysts may also develop in the third trimester **(Fig. 2)**.

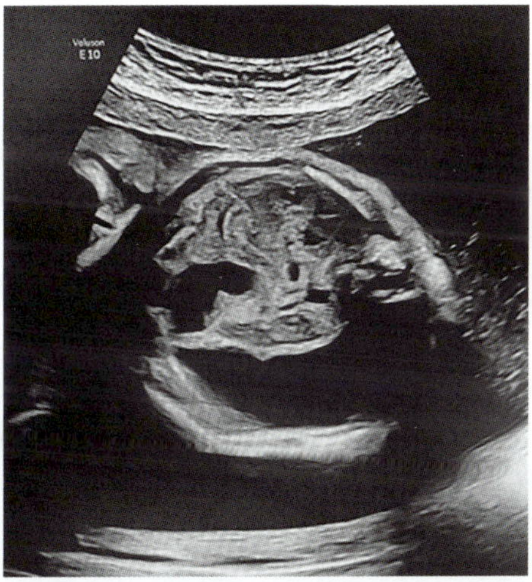

Fig. 1: Duodenal atresia.

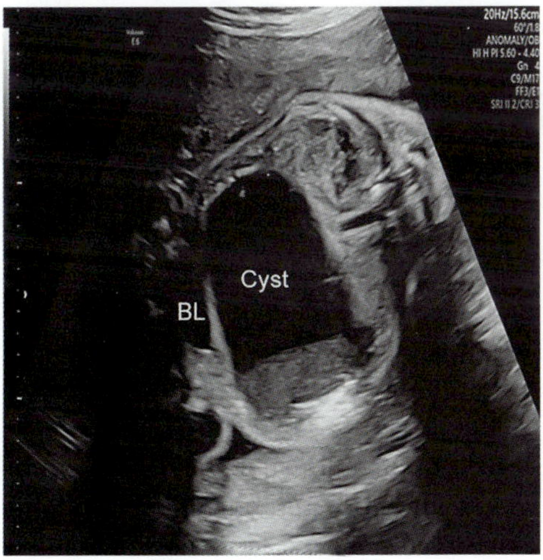

Fig. 2: Abdominal cyst.

Pyelectasis, resulting from stenosis at different points in the urinary system, can evolve from the late first trimester through delivery and into childhood.

Achondroplasia is linked to a mutation in the fibroblast growth factor receptor, but the restricted growth of long bones only becomes apparent in mid-trimester.

Some anomalies cannot be diagnosed early because the affected organ develops later in pregnancy. A good example is the Dandy-Walker variant, where the cerebellar vermis remains open until the early second trimester, making hypoplasia undetectable until then.

Agenesis of corpus callosum as well depends on the time period for appearance of normal corpus callosum **(Fig. 3)**. Schizencephaly and cerebellar hypoplasia are also late-evolving anomalies **(Figs. 4 and 5)**.

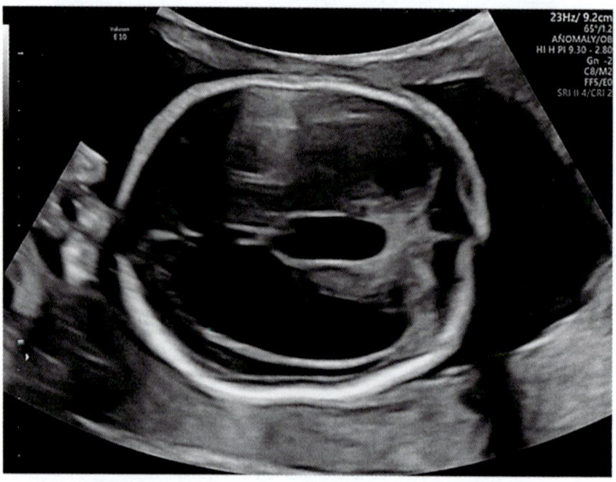

Fig. 3: Agenesis of corpous callosum.

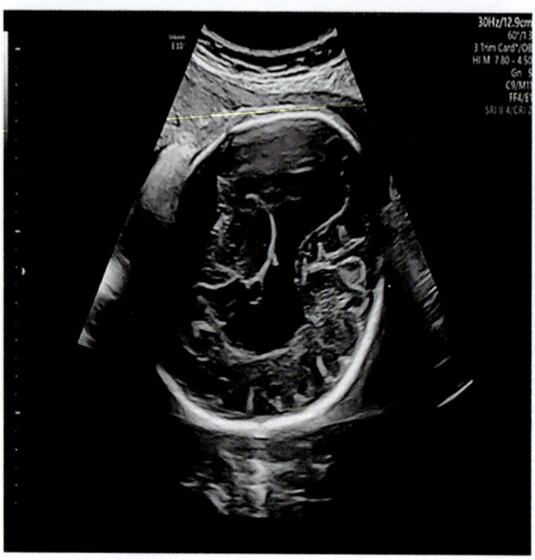

Fig. 4: Schizencephaly.

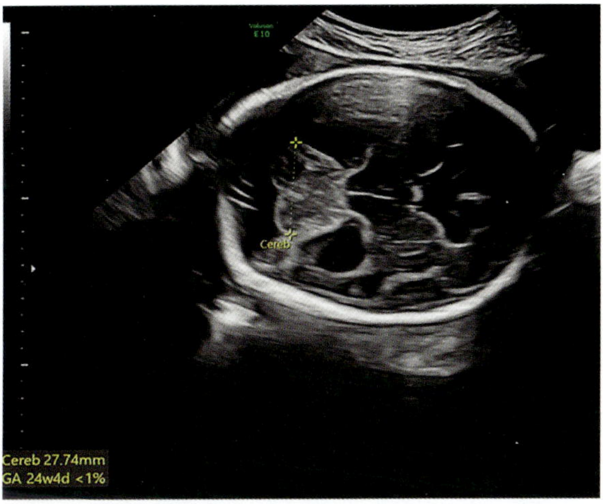

Fig. 5: Cerebellar hypoplasia.

Similarly, choroid plexus cysts, which are common in the first and early second trimesters, are considered concerning, only if they persist beyond mid-trimester.

Amniotic band syndrome is a clear example of fetal structural disruption. In one case we followed, there was a gradual reduction of the lower limb. The severity of this syndrome is thought to depend on the timing of the initial insult, emphasizing the importance of developmental timing.

Infection and hemorrhage can cause disruption of normal anatomy of brain by ACC, PACC, ventriculomegaly, hydrocephalous, porencephaly, etc.

So detailed and vigilant scanning also is required at third trimester **(Table 2)**.

Congenital Heart Diseases

Congenital heart diseases which are expressed more better in later trimester are usually evolving anomalies so should be taken care of vigilantly till the end of gestation. Sokolowski L, et al. highlighted the importance of conducting fetal echocardiography during the third trimester of pregnancy, not only in complicated pregnancies but also in normal ones.[3] It reviewed the objectives of third-trimester fetal echocardiography in various conditions, including coarctation of the aorta, premature constriction of the ductus arteriosus, increased fetal lung vascular resistance, hypoplastic left heart syndrome, dextro-transposition of the great arteries, fetal growth restriction, pregestational diabetes mellitus, and gestational diabetes mellitus.

These conditions may lead to circulatory failure that results in impaired systolic and diastolic function of myocardium, hypertrophy of myocardium, cardiomegaly and finally hydrops. These are apparent only late after the

TABLE 2: ISOUG third trimester ultrasound guideline checklist.[2]

Structure	*Parameters*	*Pathologies*
Head	Size, shape	Lissencephaly, dolichocephaly, craniosynostoses, clover-leaf skull
Brain	Symmetry of hemispheres, width of lateral ventricles, texture of cerebral cortex and parenchyma	Agyria, pachygyria, lissencephaly, ventriculomegaly, intracranial hemorrhage, vein of Galen thrombosis
Heart	Situs, size, symmetry, four chamber, outflow tract and three- vessel trachea view, cardiothoracic circumference	Pulmonary stenosis, aortic stenosis, coarctation of aorta
Chest	Diaphragm in axial and sagittal section	20% CDH in third trimester detected, hydrops
Abdomen	Fluid collection, cyst, calcification, small bowel	Small bowel >14 mm, fetal ascites, hydrops, bowel atresia
Urinary system	Renal pelvis 7 mm cut-off in 3rd trimester, renal calyces, thickness of cortex	Hydronephrosis in 60% in 3rd trimester
Placenta	Thickness, location, length	Placenta previa, placenta accreta spectrum, vasa previa, tumors
Presentations		Breech, transverse lie
Fetal growth	Biometry, Dopplers	Late SGA, Late IUGR, LGA
Amniotic fluid	Deep vertical pool	Oligohydramnios, polyhydramnios

cardiovascular system exhausted its ability adapt to the pathological process. The pressure generated by the volume of blood filling the ventricles during diastole determines the preload. It is mainly about the amount of venous blood return. It is more obvious in fetal anemia and recipient TTTS fetus. The heart adjusts by increasing the lumen of ventricle. So, these evolving dysfunctions need revaluation in later trimester also.

Unique aspects of fetal echocardiography in the third trimester:

- To focus on evaluating fetal heart function which is of paramount of importance in various conditions like multiple pregnancy, cardiomyopathies, medical disorders of pregnancy, pre-eclampsia, PIH, IUGR, any fetus heart disease with expectant management.
- Fetal heart function is necessary while monitoring impact of intrauterine therapy, impact anti-inflammatory drugs on pregnancy, hemodynamic status of fetal heart in SLE and other autoimmune diseases.
- To predict the postnatal state of newborn in case of heart ailments like; HLHS, TGA with closed foramen ovale.

- To repeat assessment of fetal heart structure in conditions where early trimester echo may miss pathologies like; aortic valve stenosis, coarctation of aorta, perimembranous and muscular VSD, total anomalous pulmonary venous return.
- Important for those pathologies which rarely can be diagnosed before third trimester like; premature ductal constriction, restricted foramen ovale, increased resistance in vascular bed of lungs.

Congenital CNS Anomalies

The prevalence of congenital CNS anomalies varies across studies, with some estimating an incidence of 3–5 per 1,000 births. Antenatal sonography plays a crucial role in evaluating the fetal brain and spine, allowing for the early detection of many CNS anomalies. However, unlike other organs, the fetal brain continues to develop throughout pregnancy, particularly in gray and white matter. The formation of certain structures depends on gestational age, making some CNS anomalies diagnosable only in the later stages of the second or third trimester. Yinon Y, et al. reviewed late of fetal central nervous system anomalies.[4] They observed 19% intracranial cysts, 15% mild ventriculomegaly, absence/dysgenesis of corpus callosum in 10%, intracerebral hemorrhage in 10%. Other anomalies included hydrocephalous, lissencephaly, craniosynostosis, periventricular pseudocysts, global brain ischemia, cerebellar hypoplasia and subopendymal nodule.

The most common anomaly in the late diagnosis group is urogenital in 55%, CNS in 18% and cardiac anomalies contributed to 14%.[2]

Late diagnosis of severe central nervous system (CNS) anomalies may result in third-trimester pregnancy termination, which poses ethical, moral, religious, and psychological challenges for parents, though it is permitted in few countries.

Indications of *late terminations* grouped into four categories:[5]

1. *Late prognosis:* Fetal prognosis could not be assessed until third trimester
2. *Late diagnosis:* Second trimester not detectable
3. *Late decision:* Though findings, diagnostic and prognostic assessment completed during second trimester
4. *Missed diagnosis:* Last trimester USG findings should have been detected earlier.

Cordier AG, et al. observed late TOP in 37 % with false-negative result from earlier USG, in 18% USG findings are not detectable before third trimester and in 40% with lethal diagnosis non palatable to life.[6] Ethical issues in termination must be dealt by all regulations of concerned geography.

Even in countries where late-term termination is not allowed, early detection of anomalies is essential. It can improve the outcomes for newborns, as some cases may require delivery at a specialized tertiary care facility. Clinicians should have enough knowledge regarding evolving pathologies and their pathogenesis, so that appropriately can be managed in all aspects.

REFERENCES

1. Yagel S, Achiron R. Developmental fetal malformations: time to change the terminology. Ultrasound Obstet Gynaecol. 1998;11:89-91.
2. ISOUG Practice Guidelines: Performance of third trimester obstetric ultrasound. Ultrasound Obstet Gynaecol. 2024;63:131-47.
3. Sokolowski L, et al. Fetal echocardiography in the third trimester of pregnancy as an essential element of modern prenatal diagnostics and perinatal care—recommendations of the Polish Society of Prenatal Cardiology 2020. Prenat Cardio. 2020. Doi:htps:// doi.org/10.5114/pcard2020.102272.
4. Yinon. Y. Late diagnosis of fetal central nervous system anomalies following a normal second trimester anatomy scan. Prenatal Diagnosis. DOI: 10.1002/pd.4163.
5. Cordier AG, et al. Evolution of third trimester pregnancy terminations in France. European J of Obst & Gynae & Reprod Biol. 2020;248:123-7.
6. Dommergues M, Benachi A, Benifla JL, des Noettes R, Dumez Y. The reasons for termination of pregnancy in the third trimester. Br J Obstet Gynaecol. 1999;106:297-303.

6

CHAPTER

Addressing Minor Markers

Karra Sahithi Reddy

INTRODUCTION

Minor markers are the ultrasound findings identified during a fetal evaluation in the mid trimester of pregnancy.[1] They are also known as soft markers. They were originally introduced to improve the detection of trisomy 21 over the age-based and serum screening strategies. Though they do not represent a structural abnormality, as there is a known association with an increased aneuploidy risk, they have importance when noted. Thus, understanding the minor markers and addressing them needs a protocol-based approach which can help in counseling and preventing unnecessary interventions.[2] The following points are to be considered while one counsels a couple when markers are detected in their unborn:

- Accuracy at which the assessment of the a-priori-risk (age risk) was calculated of the aneuploidy of interest.
- The post-test risk achieved based on results of a screening test, if performed.
- Review the identified soft marker based on validated ultrasound definitions.
- Accuracy at which the adjusted or final risk has been calculated considering the positive and negative likelihood ratios (LRs).

The following are the most widely examined markers and their USG definitions:

- Ventriculomegaly—diameter of the lateral cerebral ventricle was ≥10 mm **(Fig. 1)**.
- Increased nuchal fold—thickness was ≥6 mm **(Fig. 2)**.
- Echogenic bowel—equal echogenicity to that of bone **(Fig. 3)**
- *Mild hydronephrosis:* AP diameter of the renal pelvis >4 mm **(Fig. 4)**
- Short humerus and femur—ratio of the observed to expected length of bone (based on biparietal diameter) is <0.90, <0.92 respectively **(Fig. 5)**
- Hypoplastic nasal bone—length <0.75 MoM for the gestational age **(Fig. 6)**

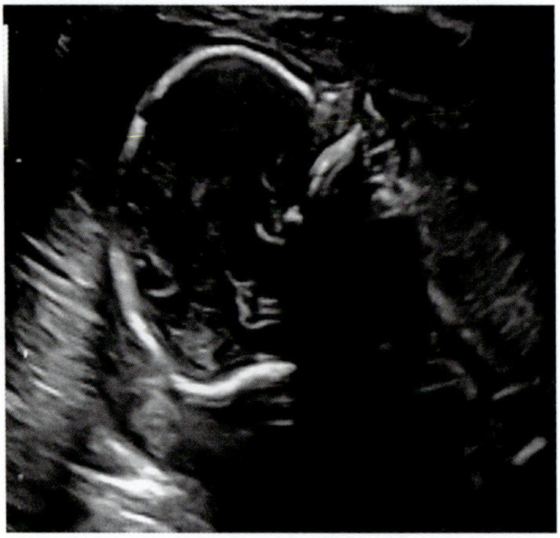

Fig. 1: Hypoplastic nasal bone.

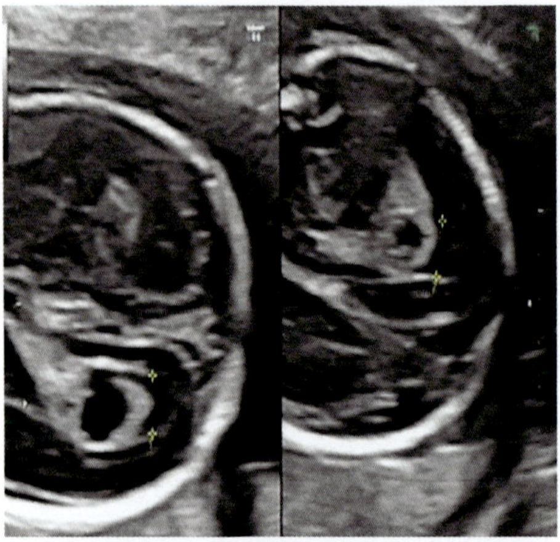

Fig. 2: Choroid plexus cyst.

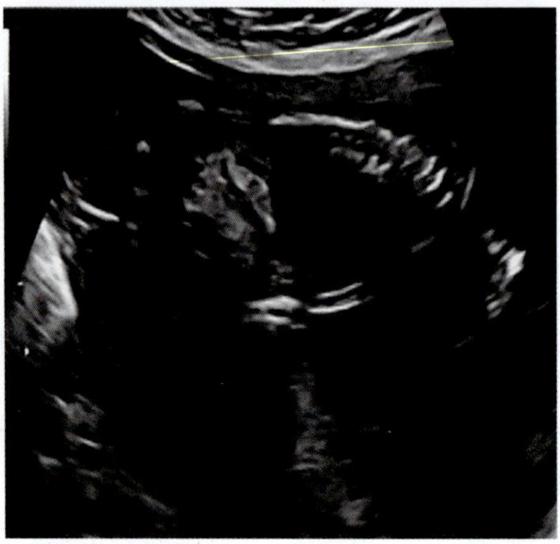

Fig. 3: Echogenic bowel.

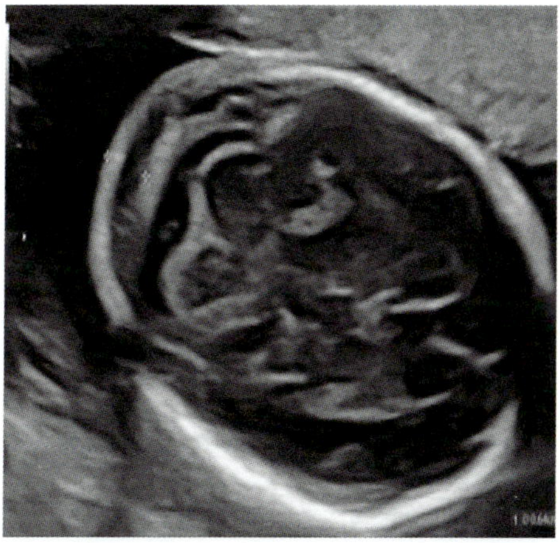

Fig. 4: Increased nuchal fold.

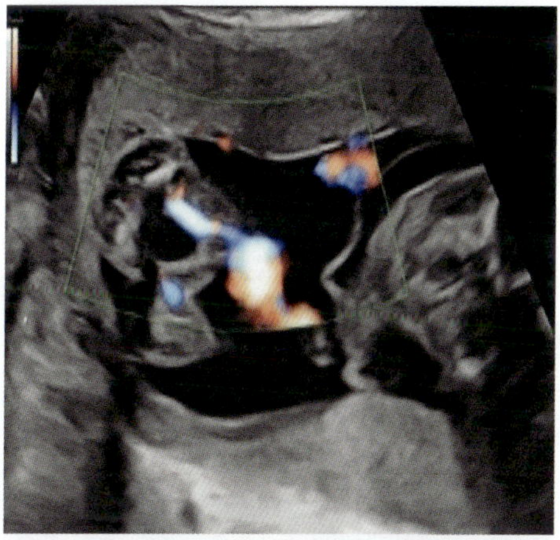

Fig. 5: Single umbilical artery.

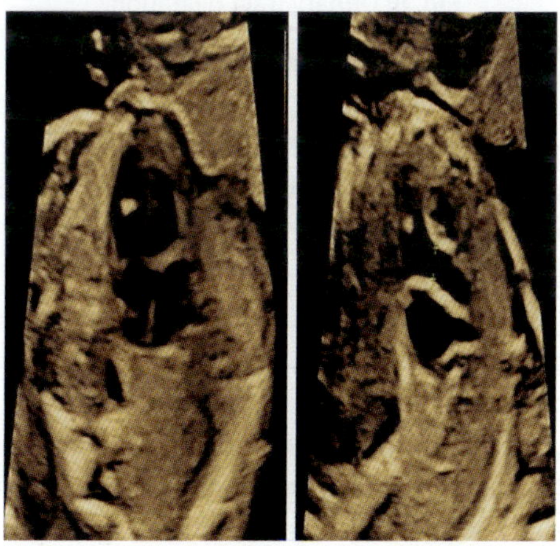

Fig. 6: Intracardiac echogenic foci.

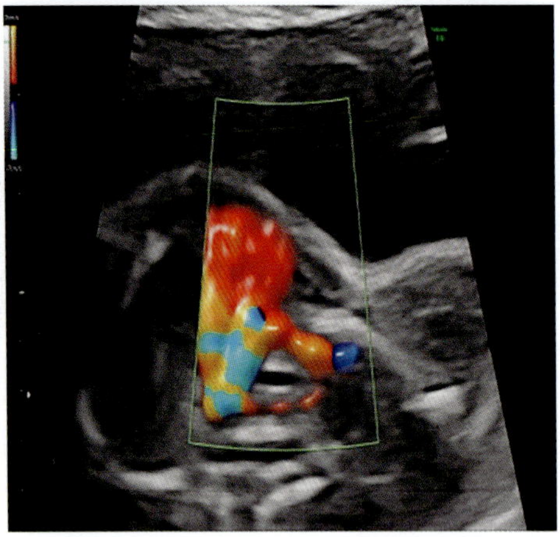

Fig. 7: Aberrant right subclavian artery.

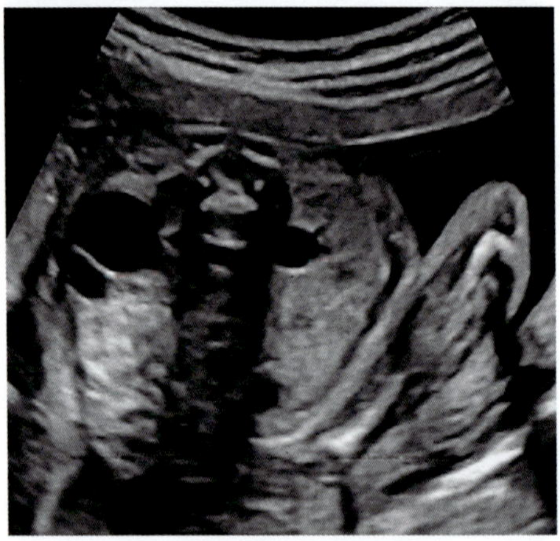

Fig. 8: Urinary tract dilatation.

- Intracardiac hyperechogenic foci—bright echogenic spot (<6 mm) seen in the cardiac chambers demonstrable in two separate planes **(Fig. 7)**.
- Aberrant right subclavian artery—the right subclavian artery which originates beyond the left subclavian artery courses behind the trachea to the right side **(Fig. 8)**.
- Choroid plexus cyst—anechoic or hypoechoic cystic areas (>2 mm) in the one or both choroid plexuses **(Fig. 9)**
- Single umbilical artery

Every mother has an age-based risk of having an aneuploidy baby. This age alone risk is "a-priori-risk". If a marker is present, then risk increases as per the LR of the marker and that is the "adjusted risk".[3] The Likelihood ratio (LR) is a statistical measurement that compares the probability of a test result

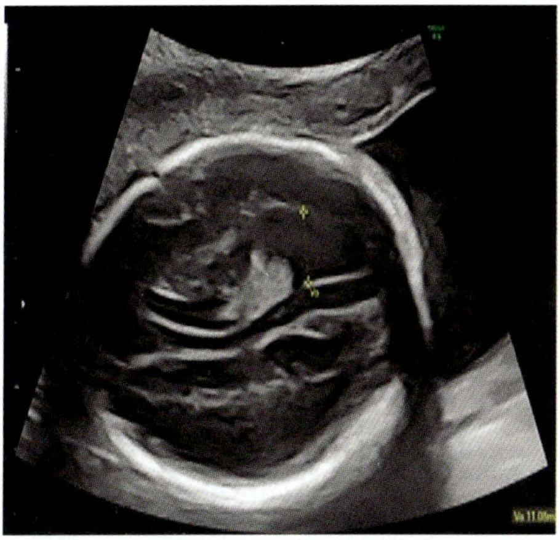

Fig. 9: Ventriculomegaly.

TABLE 1: Marker for likelihood ratio (LR).

Markers	*LR+*	*LR–*	*LR isolated marker*
EIF	5.83	0.8	0.95
Ventriculomegaly	27.5	0.94	3.8
Increased NF	23.3	0.8	3.79
Echogenic bowel	11.4	0.9	1.65
Mild hydronephrosis	7.6	0.9	1.08
Short humerus	4.8	0.7	0.78
Short femur	3.72	0.8	0.61
ARSA	21.4	0.7	3.9
Absent/hypoplastic NB	23.3	0.46	6.58

in a patient with a disease to the probability of the same result in a patient without the disease. Every soft marker has been assigned a likelihood ratio (LR) and this is used to calculate the final risk and helps in deciding about the requirement of next test **(Table 1)**.

So, addressing the minor markers depends on the "a-priori-risk", the Likelihood ratio of the marker noted, and the final new adjusted risk achieved **(Flowchart 1)**.

The a-priori-risk in most of the settings in current day practice is a first trimester combined screening test (NT scan and a biochemical test) which allocates the mother into a low-risk or high-risk group.[4] Further a Targeted Imaging for Fetal Anomalies (TIFFA) is done at 18–24 weeks. If an isolated soft marker is noted the risk will be reallocated based on the previous aneuploidy screening results along with additional risk factors for aneuploidy—such

Flowchart 1: Likelihood ratio (LR).

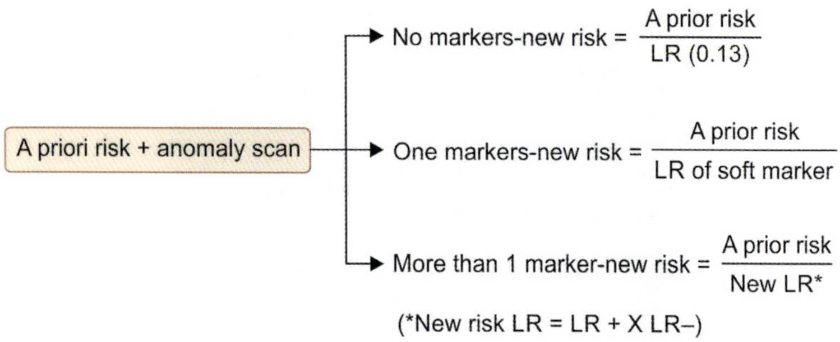

as family history and associations with non-aneuploidy conditions such as cystic fibrosis, infections. Most of the isolated markers have only a small change on the pre-test risk for trisomy 21, but with ventriculomegaly, nuchal fold thickness and ARSA there is a 3–4-fold increase in risk and with hypoplastic nasal bone a 6–7-fold increase even though they are found as isolated markers. If multiple soft markers are identified or co existing structural abnormalities are seen, the approach to evaluation should be individualized.[5]

In recent times, the relevance of soft marker findings noted during the mid-trimester fetal evaluation has changed with a cfDNA being done as a screening test because of its high sensitivity and specificity. A negative cfDNA result lowers the risk of trisomy 21 by 300-fold, so considering the reduction in the risk of having an aneuploid fetus some of the soft markers with highest positive LRs have a low relevance.[6,7]

Some of the soft markers such as ventriculomegaly, pelviectasis, short, long bones, echogenic bowel need a serial follow-up even though the fetus is labeled as a low risk or no risk fetus **(Table 2)**.

CONCLUSION

While addressing minor markers for fetal aneuploidies, it is important to convey a balanced perspective, acknowledge both the implications and need for further testing. While the presence of minor markers for fetal aneuploidies has been observed, these findings are not definitive for aneuploidy and should be interpreted within the broader context of the overall assessment. It is crucial to discuss these results with a specialist to understand the significance and explore additional diagnostic options that may recommend for a comprehensive evaluation.

Addressing minor markers not only include counseling and testing to rule out aneuploidies but also includes planning regular follow-up appointments which includes targeted imaging and monitoring which are crucial to track fetal development and promptly address any emerging concerns to optimize the outcomes.

TABLE 2: Management of fetuses with minor markers.[2]

Minor marker	*Screening*	*Management*	*Follow-up*
Absent/ hypoplastic nasal bone (or) Increased Nuchal fold thickness (or) Choroid plexus cyst	• *cfDNA negative:* None • *Serum screen negative:* Counseling for no further testing vs. noninvasive vs. invasive testing for aneuploidy • *No previous screening:* Counseling for noninvasive vs. invasive testing for aneuploidy	Routine care	Not applicable
Echogenic intracardiac foci	• *cfDNA or serum screen negative:* None • *No previous screening:* Counseling for noninvasive testing for aneuploidy	Routine care	Not applicable
Echogenic bowel	• *cfDNA or serum screen negative:* None • *No previous screening:* Counseling for noninvasive testing for aneuploidy	Evaluation for cystic fibrosis, congenital viral infection, intra-amniotic bleeding	Third-trimester ultrasound examination for reassessment and evaluation of growth
Urinary tract dilatation	• *cfDNA or serum screen negative:* None • *No previous screening:* Counseling for non-invasive testing for aneuploidy	Evaluation for persistence, with frequency of evaluation dependent on initial findings	Third-trimester ultrasound examination to determine whether postnatal pediatric urology or nephrology follow-up is needed
Short femur/ radius	• *cfDNA or serum screen negative:* None • *No previous screening:* Counseling for non-invasive testing for aneuploidy	Evaluation for skeletal dysplasia	Third-trimester ultrasound examination for reassessment and evaluation of growth
Single umbilical artery	*cfDNA or serum screen negative or no previous screening:* None	Consideration for weekly antenatal surveillance beginning at 36 0/7 week of gestation	Third-trimester ultrasound examination for evaluation of growth

Source: Prabhu M, Kuller JA, Biggio JR. Society for Maternal-Fetal Medicine. SMFM Consult Series #57: Evaluation and management of isolated soft ultrasound markers for aneuploidy in the second trimester. Am J Obstet Gynecol. 2021;225(4):B2-B15.

REFERENCES

1. Agathokleous M, Chaveeva P, Poon LC, Kosinski P, Nicolaides KH. Meta-analysis of second-trimester markers for trisomy 21. Ultrasound Obstet Gynecol. 2013;41(3):247-61. doi: 10.1002/uog.12364. Epub 2013 Jan 24. PMID: 23208748.
2. Prabhu M, Kuller JA, Biggio JR. Society for Maternal-Fetal Medicine. SMFM Consult Series#57: Evaluation and management of isolated soft ultrasound markers for aneuploidy in the second trimester. Am J Obstet Gynecol. 2021;225(4):B2-B15.
3. Benacerraf BR, Gelman R, Frigoletto FD Jr. Sonographic identification of second-trimester fetuses with Down's syndrome. N Engl J Med. 1987;317(22):1371-6. doi: 10.1056/NEJM198711263172203. PMID: 2960895.
4. Weerakkody Y, Campos A, Yap J, et al. Antenatal soft markers on ultrasound. Reference article, Radiopaedia.org (Accessed on 20th Sept 2024). https://doi.org/10.53347/rID-13183.
5. Gil MM, Accurti V, Santacruz B, Plana MN, Nicolaides KH. Analysis of cell-free DNA in maternal blood in screening for aneuploidies: updated meta-analysis. Ultrasound Obstet Gynecol. 2017;50(3):302-14. doi: 10.1002/uog.17484. Epub 2017 Jul 27. Update in: Ultrasound Obstet Gynecol. 2019;53(6):734-42. doi: 10.1002/uog.20284. PMID: 28397325.
6. Society for Maternal-Fetal Medicine (SMFM). Electronic address: pubs@smfm.org; Norton ME, Biggio JR, Kuller JA, Blackwell SC. The role of ultrasound in women who undergo cell-free DNA screening. Am J Obstet Gynecol. 2017;216(3):B2-B7. doi: 10.1016/j.ajog.2017.01.005. Epub 2017 Jan 17. PMID: 28108156.
7. Reddy UM, Abuhamad AZ, Levine D, Saade GR; Fetal Imaging Workshop Invited Participants. Fetal imaging: Executive Summary of a joint Eunice Kennedy Shriver National Institute of Child Health and Human Development, Society for Maternal-Fetal Medicine, American Institute of Ultrasound in Medicine, American College of Obstetricians and Gynecologists, American College of Radiology, Society for Pediatric Radiology, and Society of Radiologists in Ultrasound Fetal Imaging Workshop. J Ultrasound Med. 2014;33(5):745-57. doi: 10.7863/ultra.33.5.745. PMID: 24764329.

7 CHAPTER

Mid-Trimester Anomaly Scan

Chandrakant Garg

INTRODUCTION

The mid-trimester anomaly ultrasound (MTAS), also known as the second-trimester anatomy scan, is a routine examination that plays a pivotal role in ensuring the well-being of the developing fetus, typically performed between 18 and 22 weeks of gestation. Its primary aim is to assess fetal anatomy and detect any anomalies, though detection rates may vary depending on factors such as operator training, machine settings, amniotic fluid volume, and fetal position.

All pregnant women should be offered a mid-trimester anomaly scan as part of routine antenatal care. The mother should be counseled for the benefits and limitations of the routine mid-trimester anomaly scan. This scan evaluates cardiac activity, gestational age/fetal size, fetal anatomy, placental position/ appearance, cervical length and amniotic fluid volume. The scan also serves as a baseline for comparing fetal growth in later scans.

Prenatal diagnosis significantly reduces perinatal mortality and morbidity, as well as maternal morbidity. It enables earlier and less psychologically traumatic medical termination of pregnancy when necessary. Additionally, it helps reduce potential complications associated with continuing pregnancy and prevents unnecessary cesarean sections for fetus with lethal anomalies detected too late.

GUIDELINES FOR EXAMINATION

Fetal Biometry and Wellbeing

Fetal biometry, including measurements of biparietal diameter (BPD), head circumference (HC), abdominal circumference (AC), and femur length (FL), is routinely performed to assess fetal size. Dating should be checked. If the fetus has not been previously dated, HC or a combination of HC and FL can be used for dating after 14 weeks of gestation.

Biparietal diameter (BPD) is measured using calipers placed outer-to-outer. Key landmarks are symmetrical hemispheres, the interruption of the falx cerebri by the cavum septum pellucidum (CSP), and the cerebellum not being visible.

Head circumference (HC) **(Fig. 1A)** can be measured BPD plane using the ellipse approach or derived from biparietal diameter (BPD) and occipitofrontal diameter (OFD).

Abdominal circumference (AC) **(Fig. 1B)** is measured in a transverse section of the fetal abdomen, ideally circular, with the fetal spine positioned at 3 or 9 o'clock. AC can be measured using the ellipse approach or derived from anteroposterior and transverse abdominal diameters. Key landmarks for optimal AC imaging include a circular fetal abdomen, the umbilical vein at the portal sinus level with visible stomach and single rib on either side. The kidneys should not be visualized in the AC section.

Femur length (FL) **(Fig. 1C)** is measured with both ends of the ossified diaphysis. The longest axis of the diaphysis is measured with an insonation angle between 45° and 90°. Calipers are placed at the ends of the diaphysis, excluding the distal femoral epiphysis if visible.

Estimated fetal weight (EFW) is calculated by using the Hadlock's formula since it appears to be the most stable mathematically, and its use is recommended in most clinical scenarios.

Amniotic fluid assessment ***(Fig. 2):*** The volume of amniotic fluid surrounding the baby is a crucial indicator of fetal well-being and can significantly influence pregnancy outcomes. During an anomaly scan, the deepest vertical pool (DVP) measurement is preferred. A DVP of ≤2 cm indicates low fluid

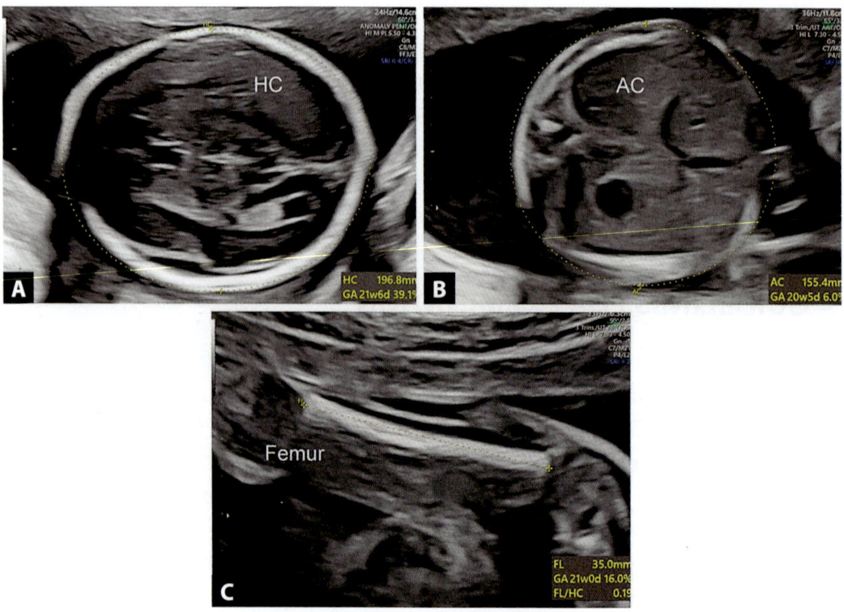

Figs. 1A to C: Standard fetal biometry. Sonographic measurements of: (A) Head circumference (HC); (B) Abdominal circumference (AC); and (C) Femur length (FL).

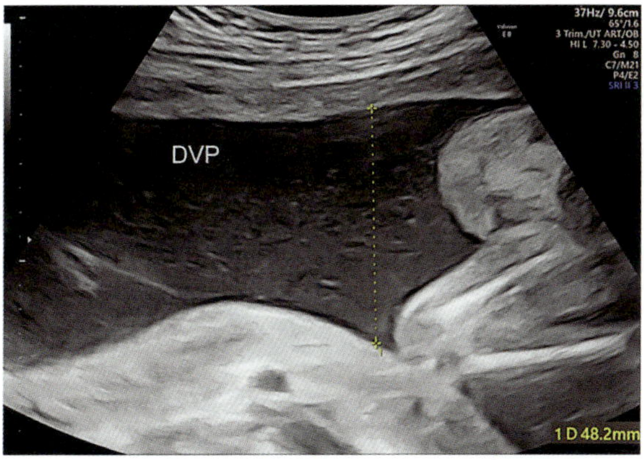

Fig. 2: Amniotic fluid assessment (DVP).

(oligohydramnios), 2–8 cm is considered normal, and >8 cm suggests high fluid (polyhydramnios).

Detailed fetal anatomy check: A thorough examination to identify any developmental abnormalities. For the mid-trimester, a basic fetal anatomical survey should meet minimum requirements. This includes:

HEAD AND BRAIN

The basic skull examination should assess size, shape, integrity, and bone density. The skull should normally appear oval in shape without any focal protrusions.

Abnormalities such as Acrania, encephalocele, abnormal skull shape (strawberry, lemon-shaped skull) and poor skull mineralization (osteogenesis imperfecta and hypophosphatasia) can be detected.

The brain examination involves mainly by two axial planes (Transventricular and Transcerebellar plane).

Transventricular Plane **(Fig. 3A)**—This plane demonstrates midline falx, cavum septi pellucidi (CSP), lateral ventricles (including the choroid plexus). The frontal horns (anterior portion) appear as two comma-shaped, fluid-filled structures, separated medially by the CSP, a fluid-filled cavity. The CSP should always be visualized between 18 and 37 weeks of gestation. An abnormal CSP may be associated with brain abnormalities such as holoprosencephaly, agenesis of the corpus callosum, severe hydrocephaly, and septo-optic dysplasia.

The posterior portion of the lateral ventricles includes the atrium, which is typically measured at the level of the parieto-occipital sulcus. In a normal fetus, the atrium should measure up to 10 mm in transverse diameter.

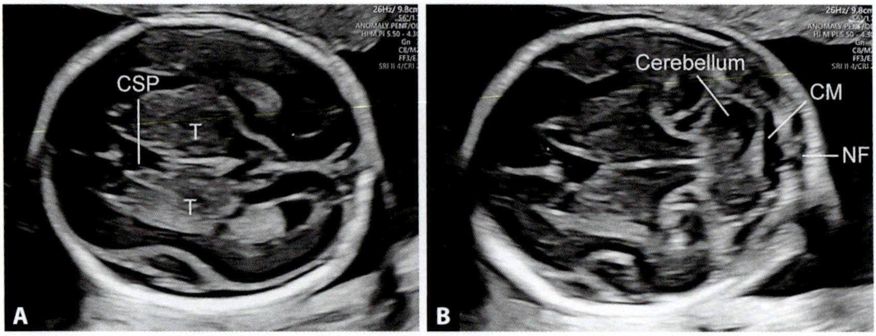

Figs. 3A and B: Transverse views of the fetal head, demonstrating standard transventricular (A) and transcerebellar (B) planes. Cavum septum pellucidum (CSP); Thalamus (T); Cisterna magna (CM); Nuchal fold thickness (NF).

Transcerebellar Plane (Fig. 3B)

This plane is located inferior to the biparietal diameter (BPD) plane and is obtained by tilting the probe backward into the posterior fossa. It is correctly visualized when the thalami, cavum septum pellucidum, and cerebellum are seen together. The cerebellum appears as a dumbbell-shaped structure with symmetrical lobes, and the central vermis is slightly more echogenic than the lateral lobes.

The transcerebellar diameter (TCD), measured as the widest distance across the cerebellum perpendicular to the falx, correlates with gestational age up to 20 weeks.

The cisterna magna is measured from the posterior margin of the cerebellar vermis to the inner surface of the occipital bone in the midline, with normal values ranging from 2 to 10 mm during the second and third trimesters.

The nuchal fold, measured from the outer skin line to the outer bone at the midline, is considered normal if it is less than 6 mm up to 22 weeks of gestation.

FACE

Early detection of facial abnormalities can facilitate the diagnosis of multiple syndromes, allowing for appropriate parental counseling and optimal fetal care. Fetal face evaluation includes the midsagittal facial profile **(Fig. 4B)** to check normalcy of fetal face and nasal bone. The modified coronal (frontal) view **(Fig. 4A)** for both orbits, lens, nose, lips and intact palate **(Figs. 4C and D)**.

Abnormality like flat face, retrognathia, absent nasal bone, cleft lip and palate, hypo- and hypertelorism can be detected by using these planes.

NECK

The neck should appear cylindrical without any protuberances, masses, or fluid collections. Any obvious neck masses, such as cystic hygromas, goiter, or teratomas, should be documented **(Fig. 5)**.

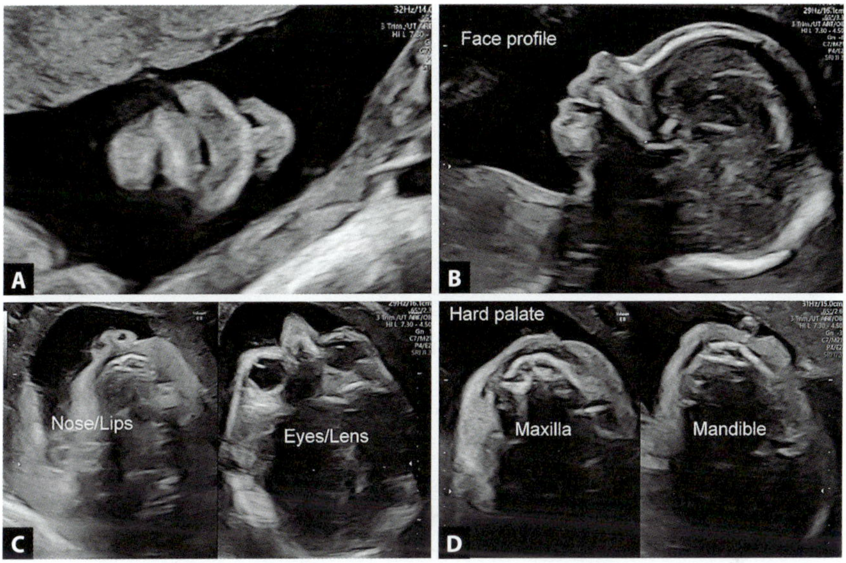

Figs. 4A to D: Ultrasound imaging of the fetal face. (A) The mouth, lips and nose are typically evaluated in a coronal view; (B) Midsagittal facial profile view; (C) Both fetal orbits should appear symmetrical and intact, with eyes separated by approximately the diameter of one orbit; (D) Intact hard palate (maxilla).

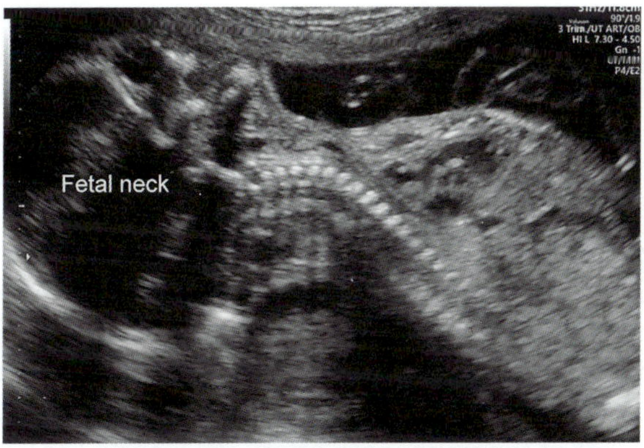

Fig. 5: Fetal neck and cervical spine.

THORAX

The thorax has a regular shape with a smooth transition to the abdomen and the ribs should have normal curvature without deformities. The shape of the thorax, the ribs, and the homogeneous echogenicity of both lungs can be assessed using axial views. The integrity of the diaphragm can be examined in either the sagittal or coronal view. The diaphragm appears as a hypoechoic line separating the thoracic and abdominal organs **(Figs. 6A and B)**.

Abnormalities such as mediastinal shift, lung masses, pleural effusions, and diaphragmatic hernia can be detected.

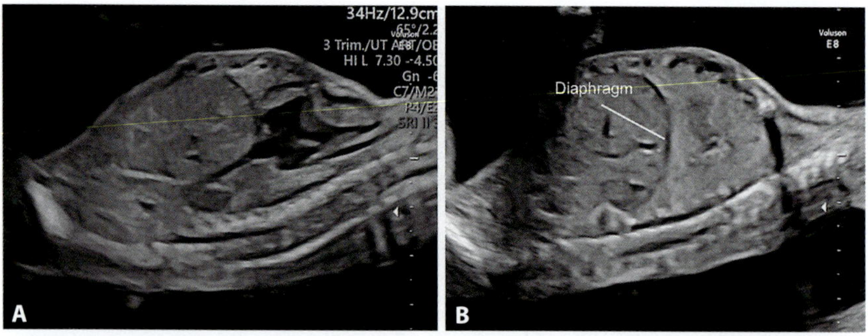

Figs. 6A and B: Sagittal section of thorax showing transition (A) and diaphragm (B).

HEART

Heart examination begins with assessing situs **(Fig. 7A)**, position, axis, and rhythm. Anatomical evaluation includes the four-chamber view **(Fig. 7B)**, outflow tract views, and the three-vessel view, aiming to detect congenital heart disease during the mid-trimester scan. A normal heart is on the left side of chest, taking up no more than one-third of the chest area, with an axis of about 45±20° to the left side. The fetal heart rate ranges from 120–160 bpm.

In addition to the four-chamber view, routine screening should assess the left ventricular outflow tract **(Fig. 7C)** and right ventricular outflow tract **(Fig. 7D)**, which cross each other (Crossover) as they exit the ventricles. This improves detection of malformations like tetralogy of Fallot, transposition of the great arteries, and double-outlet right ventricle. The three-vessel view **(Fig. 7E)** and three-vessel-trachea views **(Fig. 7F)** help to identify outflow tract and aortic arch anomalies.

The basic fetal cardiac planes with color doppler **(Fig. 8)** include the following: The four-chamber view **(Fig. 8A)** assesses symmetry, size, and unidirectional valve flow. The LVOT **(Fig. 8B)** visualizes smooth aortic outflow, while the RVOT **(Fig. 8C)** demonstrates pulmonary outflow with bifurcation of the pulmonary artery. The three-vessel view (3VV) **(Fig. 8D)** shows alignment of the pulmonary artery (PA), aorta (Ao), and superior vena cava (SVC) with forward flow, and the three-vessel-trachea view (3VT) **(Fig. 8E)** highlights continuous flow in the ductal and aortic arches toward the descending aorta. Additionally, the NRSA (normal right subclavian artery) **(Fig. 8F)** view confirms the normal origin and course of the right subclavian artery from the aortic arch.

ABDOMEN

The abdominal situs should be determined. The fetal stomach must be identified in its normal position on the left side. From left to right, the stomach, umbilical vein, and gallbladder should be visualized. The fetal

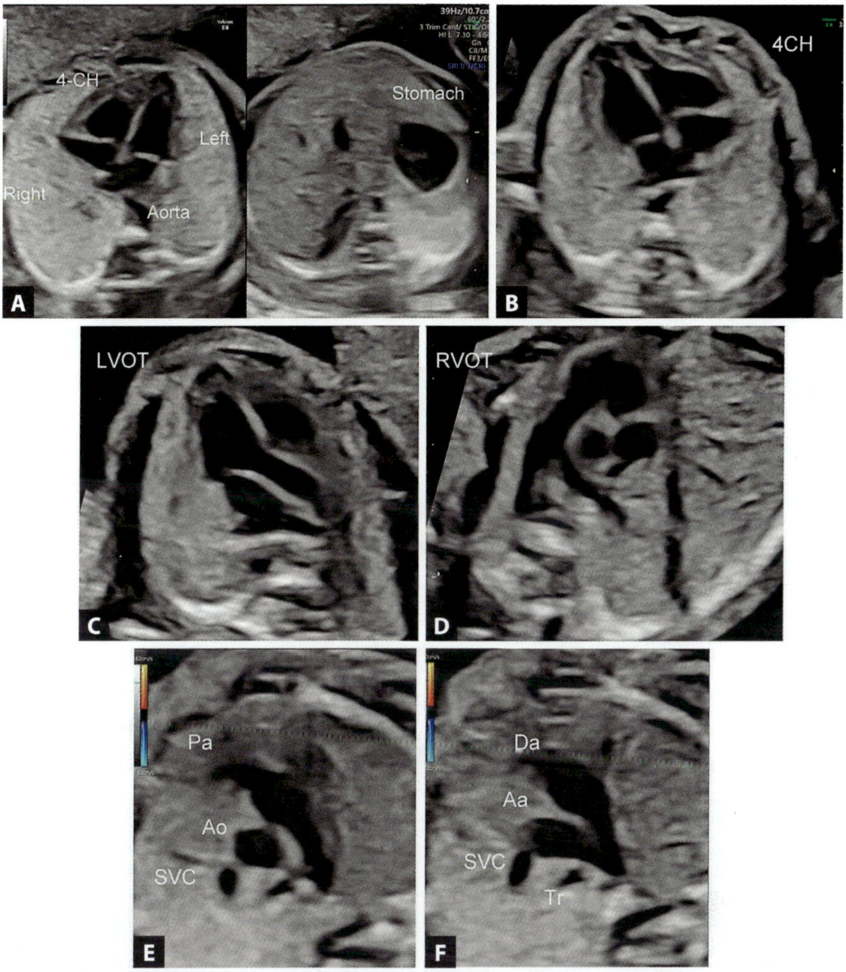

Figs. 7A to F: (A) Scan planes for mid-trimester fetal cardiac screening. The four-chamber view (4CV) (B); Left ventricular outflow tract (LVOT) (C) (arrow); Right ventricular outflow tract (RVOT) (D); Three-vessel view (E); Three-vessel-trachea view (F) [pulmonary artery (Pa), ascending aorta (Ao) and right superior vena cava (SVC)] and three-vessels-and-trachea view (E) [ductal arch (Da), aortic arch (Aa), right superior vena cava (SVC) and trachea (Tr)] are documented in addition to the 4CV.

umbilical cord insertion site **(Fig. 9A)** should be examined for any evidence of a ventral wall defect. Any abnormal fluid around the bowel suggestive of ascites. If bowels are bright and echogenicity equal to bone, one should think for hyperechogenic bowel (HEB).

The two most common congenital abdominal wall defects are omphalocele and gastroschisis. *Omphalocele* appears as an outpouching of the abdominal wall, covered by an inner membrane of parietal peritoneum. *Gastroschisis* is characterized by a full-thickness defect in the abdominal

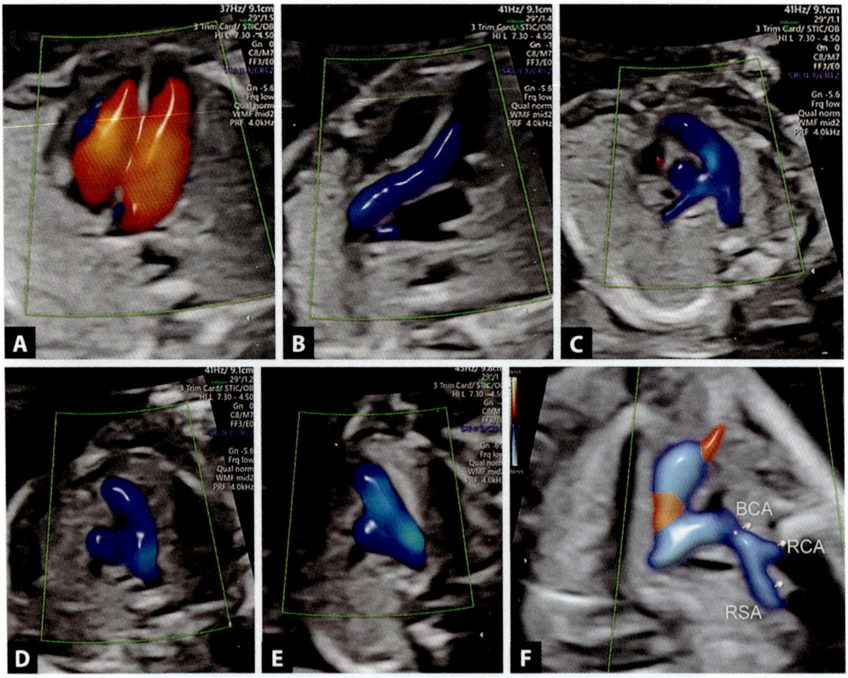

Figs. 8A to F: Fetal heart with color Doppler: (A) The four-chamber view; (B) Left ventricular outflow tract (LVOT); (C) Right ventricular outflow tract (RVOT); (D) Three-vessel view; (E) Three-vessel-trachea view; (F) Normal right subclavian artery (NRSA).

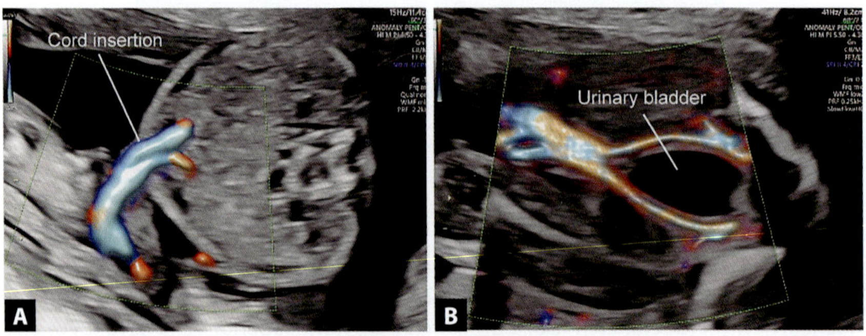

Figs. 9A and B: Ultrasound imaging of the fetal cord insertion site (A) and urinary bladder with two umbilical arteries (B).

wall that allows for evisceration of the fetal abdominal contents. Other Abnormalities like small/absent stomach bubble, double bubble appearance can be detected.

KIDNEYS AND BLADDER

Both kidneys to be check in axial, coronal, and sagittal planes. Normal kidneys, along with the adrenal glands, are located on either side of the spine, just below the level of the fetal stomach. In the early weeks, the kidneys appear

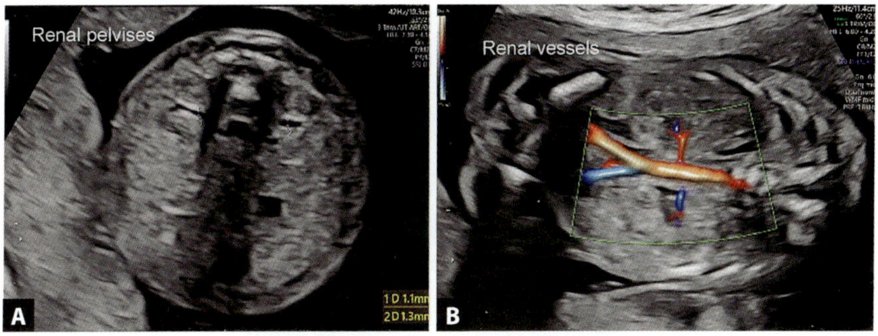

Figs. 10A and B: Axial view of kidneys with renal pelvises AP diameter (A) and coronal views of kidneys with renal vessels (B).

echogenic but gradually become hypoechoic compared to the adjacent bowel and liver. Axial plane **(Fig. 10A)** is used to measure anteroposterior diameter of renal pelvises. A renal pelvis ≥5 mm is a soft marker for T21, renal pelvis >7 mm requires reassessment in the third trimester. Both renal vessels can be visualized using the color Doppler **(Fig. 10B)**.

The fetal bladder **(Fig. 9B)** should visualize between two umbilical arteries, demonstrates 3 vessels cord. Fetal ureters are typically not visible on antenatal scans unless they are dilated. An enlarged bladder (megacystis) or persistent absence of the bladder needs further assessment.

SPINE

The basic fetal spine examination should include transverse, sagittal, and coronal views. Evaluation of the spine depends on the fetal position; however, a longitudinal view should always be obtained, as it may reveal other spinal malformations, including vertebral abnormalities and sacral agenesis.

In the sagittal plane, the ossification centers of the vertebral bodies and posterior arches form two parallel lines that converge at the sacrum. During the second and third trimesters of gestation, the conus medullaris is typically located at the level of L2 to L3. The integrity of the neural canal is inferred from the regular disposition of the ossification centers of the spine and the presence of soft tissue covering the spine **(Figs. 11A to C)**.

Spinal abnormalities like open spina bifida, kyphoscoliosis, hemivertebrae, tethered cord can be detected.

LIMBS AND EXTREMITIES

The presence of both arms, hands, legs, and feet should be documented systematically. All four limbs should be examined for long bone presence, symmetry, shape, size, alignment, position, and movement. Most prenatal-onset skeletal dysplasias present with relative disproportion in skeletal measurements **(Figs. 12A to C)**.

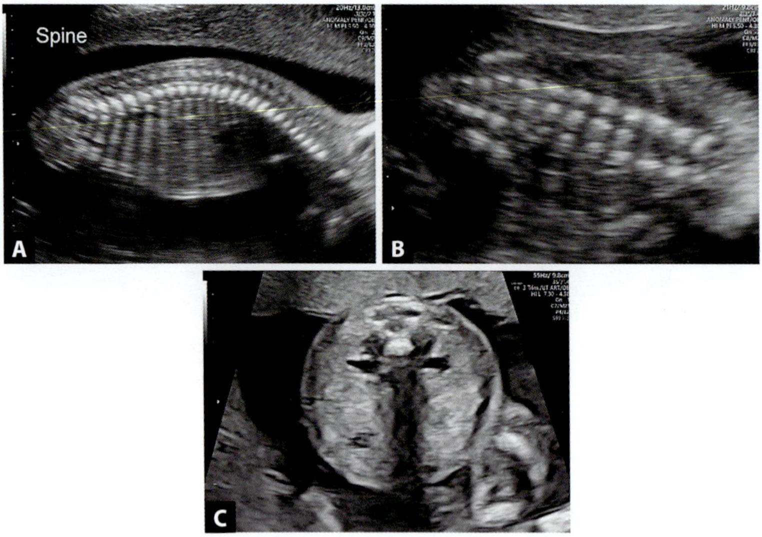

Figs. 11A to C: Longitudinal (A); Coronal (B); and Axial (C) views of the spine including a clearly visible intact skin over the spine.

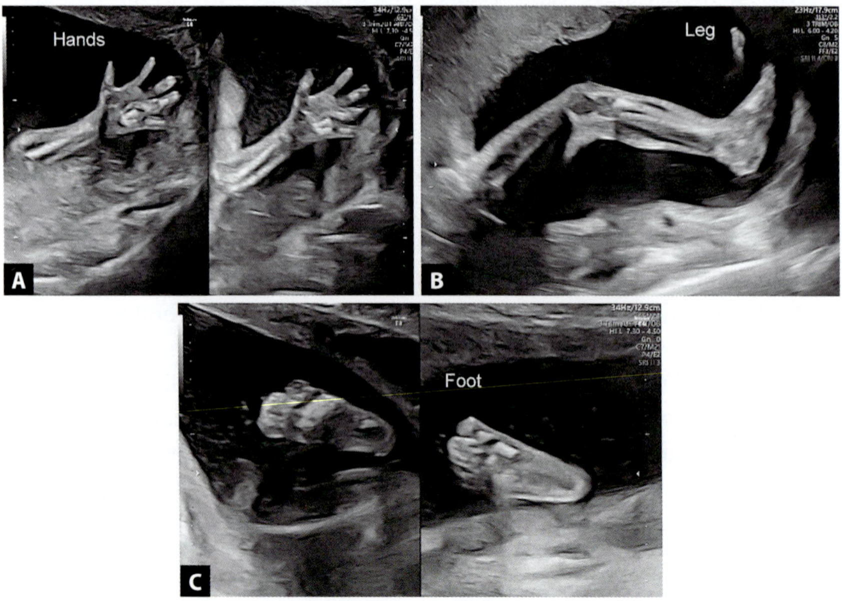

Figs. 12A to C: Image of the fetal upper (A), lower (B) extremities and foot (C).

GENITALIA

Pre-Conception and Pre-Natal Diagnostic Techniques (PCPNDT) law does not allow us to determine fetal sex in the routine mid-trimester scan.

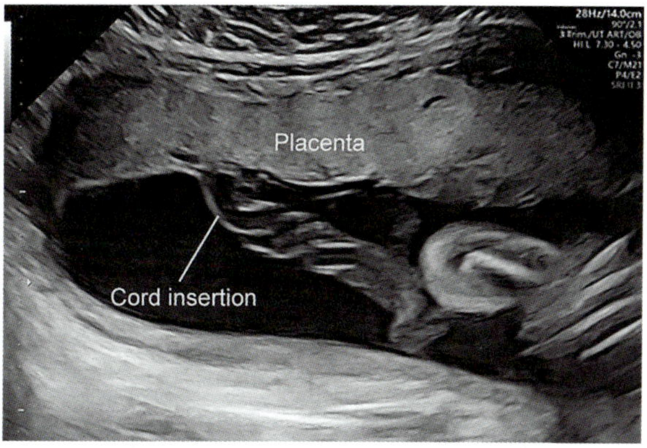

Fig. 13: Placenta and cord insertion on placental side.

Placental Assessment

The placental location, its relation to the internal cervical os (usually via transabdominal imaging), and appearance should be assessed. Abnormal findings may include hemorrhage, multiple cysts (seen in triploidy), or placental masses like chorioangioma. If the lower placental edge reaches or overlaps the internal os, follow-up in the third trimester is recommended. Suggested cut-offs for placental migration are 5 mm (anterior) and 15.5 mm (posterior) from the os, using transvaginal imaging **(Fig. 13)**.

Cord Insertion

In about 80% of cases, the umbilical cord inserts in the center of the placenta, paracentral in 12%, and marginal (within 2 cm of the edge) in 5–8%. Velamentous insertion, where the umbilical vessels insert into the membranes, occurs in 1% and may be linked to vasa previa and FGR.

Cervical Assessment

The cervix is typically evaluated through a transabdominal scan but, when possible, transvaginal cervical length (CL) measurement should be performed during the mid-trimester scan for preterm birth screening, with additional consent from the woman. A short CL (<25 mm), especially before 24 weeks, is strongly linked to preterm birth **(Fig. 14)**.

CONCLUSION

The mid-trimester fetal anomaly scan is a crucial component of prenatal care, providing essential information about fetal anatomy and well-being. By assessing various structures and systems, including the head/brain, thorax/heart, abdomen, spine, kidneys, and extremities, we can identify potential anomalies. Early detection allows for timely intervention, parental counseling,

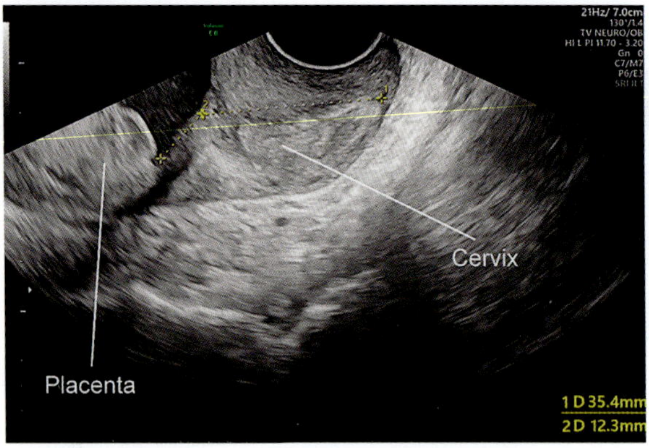

Fig. 14: Cervical length and placental position should be determined in relation to the maternal cervix.

and the planning of appropriate care strategies. This scan not only enhances fetal monitoring but also contributes to improved outcomes for both the mother and the fetus. Therefore, it is essential that all pregnant individuals be offered this important examination as part of routine antenatal care.

SUGGESTED READING

1. Dias T, Arcangeli T, Bhide A, Napolitano R, Mahsud-Dornan S, Thilaganathan B. First-trimester ultrasound determination of chorionicity in twin pregnancy. Ultrasound Obstet Gynecol 2011; 38: 530-2.
2. ISUOG-Practice-Guidelines-routine-mid-trimester-fetal-ultrasound 2022;59:840–56, Published online in Wiley Online Library (wileyonlinelibrary.com). DOI: 10.1002/uog.24888
3. Medley N, Poljak B, Mammarella S, Alfirevic Z. Clinical guidelines for prevention and management of preterm birth: a systematic review. BJOG. 2018;125:1361-9.
4. Preterm Labour and Birth. NICE Guideline, No. 25. National Institute for Health and Care Excellence: London; 2019.
5. Salomon LJ, Alfirevic Z, Da Silva Costa F, Deter RL, Figueras F, Ghi T, Glanc P, Khalil A, Lee W, Napolitano R, Papageorghiou A, Sotiriadis A, Stirnemann J, Toi A, Yeo G. ISUOG Practice Guidelines: ultrasound assessment of fetal biometry and growth. Ultrasound Obstet Gynecol. 2019;53:715-23.

8

CHAPTER

Ready Reckoner on Intrapartum USG: A DIY Manual

Bharani Vijayaragavan, Malvika Jain

INTRODUCTION

Ultrasound has come to stay in an obstetrician's armamentarium from the follicle to the fetus stage. Having a tool that accurately predicts the mode of delivery would be a dream for every obstetrician. Ultrasound in labor has been in practice for many years and helps in precise and reproducible measurement of the descent of the fetal head and the progress of labor. It can predict the likelihood of achieving a vaginal delivery, solving two problems. Firstly, removing the subjectivity of clinical assessment and secondly, providing confidence to the operator when an attempt at operative vaginal delivery is warranted. Albeit the growing body of evidence, ultrasound in active labor is not widely used in obstetric units for fear of a long-learning curve. In this article, we would like to highlight the practical aspects of intrapartum USG, how to take measurements, and its interpretation for easy learning and clinical use.[1]

HOW TO PREPARE THE PROBE?

Intrapartum USG can be used to assess the position, station, rotation, degree of rotation, asynclitism, and caput and molding of the fetal head. A regular 3.5 MHz curved transducer can be used for transabdominal and transperineal measurements. For transperineal measurement, the probe can be covered using a transparent "Safe Hands" glove with scan gel smeared inside and outside the cover.[2]

TRANSABDOMINAL PROBE

Digital examination has significant limitations when determining fetal head position and studies have found that clinicians erroneously assign occipito-posterior position in almost 50% of cases. The fetal head position can be readily assessed transabdominally by locating the fetal spine and the occiput. The probe is placed transversely on the suprapubic area. A transverse midline echo of the corpus callosum identifies an occiput transverse position **(Fig. 1)**. Visualization of the fetal orbits above the

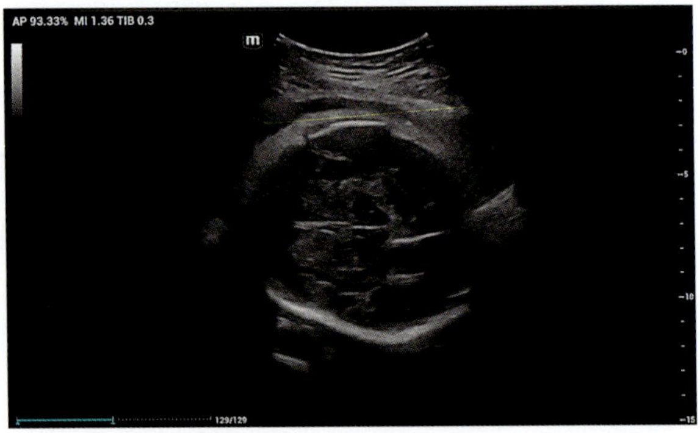

Fig. 1: Transverse position.

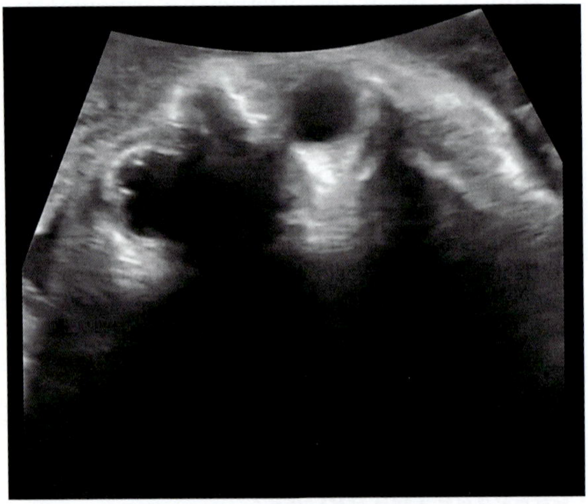

Fig. 2: Occiput-posterior position.

symphysis pubis positively confirms an occiput posterior position **(Fig. 2)**. Once occipito-posterior is confirmed, the next step is to identify if the spine is anterior or posterior. If the spine is anterior, the probability of the head rotating and delivering is greater, and persistent occipito-posterior is more often seen when the spine is posterior. A chin-on-chest appearance with an anteriorly visible fetal heart predicts an increased likelihood of a fetal head **(Fig. 3)**. Occiput spinal angle is another measurement taken in the sagittal plane as the angle between two tangential lines to the occipital bone and the vertebral body of the first cervical spine is measured three times and the mean is taken **(Fig. 4)**. A more obtuse angle predicts the success of vaginal delivery.[3]

Asynclitism is easily detected sonographically by placing the ultrasonic beam at right angles to the midline echo. In anterior asynclitism, the

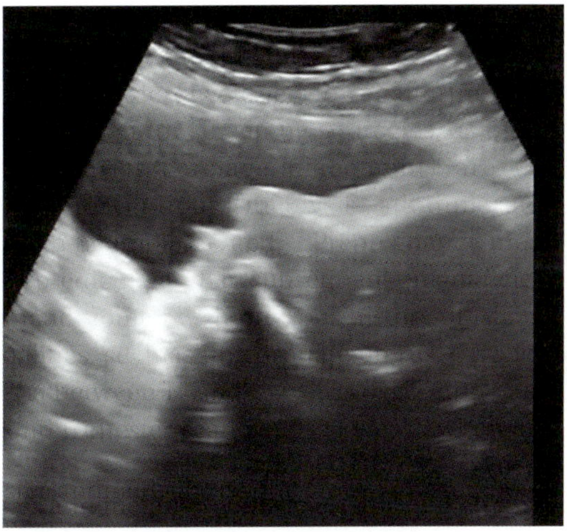

Fig. 3: Chin-chest position.

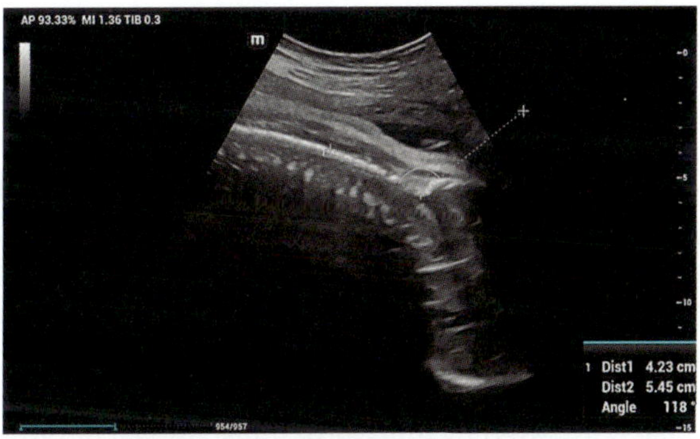

Fig. 4: Occiput-spinal angle.

anterior orbit ("squint sign" or "Malvasi's sign 1"), the north thalamus sunset ("thalamus sunset" or "Malvasi's sign 2"), and the north cerebellum sunset ("cerebellum sunset" or "Malvasi's sign 3") are visualized. In posterior asynclitism, the posterior orbit, the south thalamus, and the south cerebellum sunset are visualized.[4]

TRANSPERINEAL PROBE

Several transperineal ultrasound methods have been proposed to describe fetal head descent or station. Because of the difficulty of identifying the ischial spines on ultrasound, it is not possible to measure fetal head descent directly concerning the ischial spines as would be conventionally assessed when performing digital examination. Two easy and most commonly used methods to assess fetal head descent are described below.

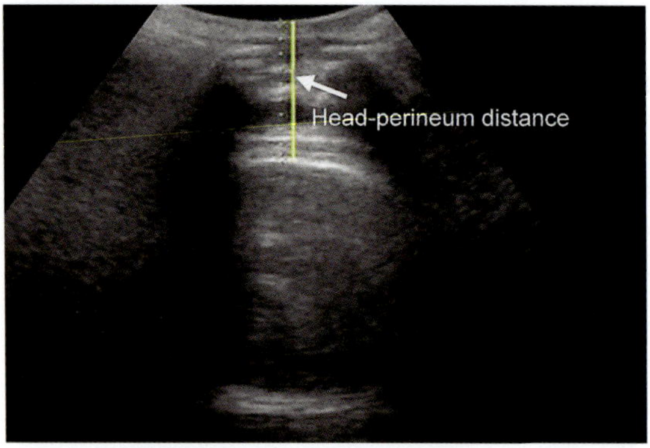

Fig. 5: Head-perineum distance.

A simple method to measure the descent of the fetal head using intrapartum ultrasound is to place the transducer transversely just above the posterior fourchette and measure the shortest distance from the transducer edge to the fetal skull which is the head-perineum distance, measured by calculating the shortest distance from the perineal skin surface to the outmost bony limit of the fetal skull in a transverse view. A shorter head-perineum distance **(Fig. 5)** was significantly associated with a shorter time to delivery and a head-perineal distance of 30 mm or less at full dilatation favors vaginal delivery. It is relatively safe for women with ruptured membranes too. Applying too much pressure must be avoided to make precise measurements.

The direction of the head **(Figs. 6A to C)** along the curve of Carus can also be looked for when serial images are taken and can be used as a tool to predict the success of operative vaginal delivery when a head is in an upward direction with a rotation <45°.

Midline angle is assessed by transverse transperineal ultrasound and may help to decide whether assisted vaginal delivery can be attempted safely. The echogenic line interposed between the two cerebral hemispheres is considered as midline and the angle between this line and the anteroposterior axis of the maternal pelvis is measured.

The angle of progression is an accurate and reproducible method of assessing the descent of the fetal head in labor **(Fig. 7)**. It is the angle between the longitudinal axis of the pubic bone and a line joining the lowest edge of the pubis to the lowest convexity of the fetal skull. An angle of progression greater than 126° predicts an easy and successful vacuum or spontaneous vaginal delivery.

In the midsagittal plane, the pubic symphysis is seen as an oblong, irregular, echogenic structure. An imaginary line originating from the caudal end of the symphysis pubis, perpendicular to its long axis is drawn and is called an infrapubic line. A line 3 cm away from this is taken as an interspinal line corresponding to 0 station. The level of the outer table of the fetal skull from this line represents the head station **(Fig. 8)**.

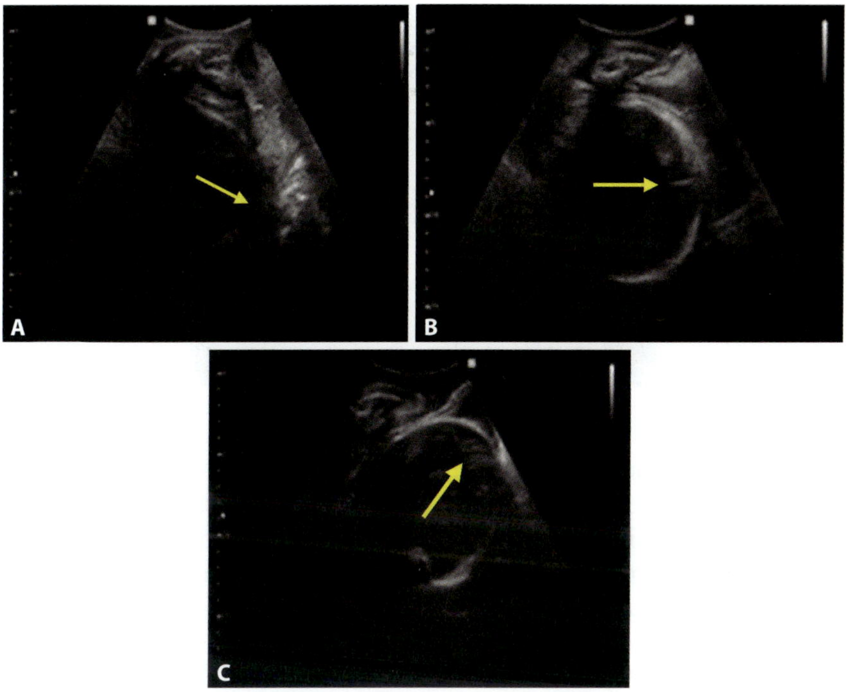

Figs. 6A to C: The direction of the fetal head.

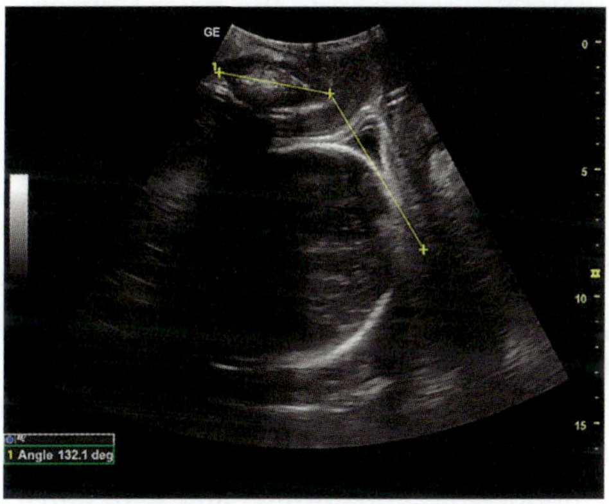

Fig. 7: Angle of progression.

USES OF INTRAPARTUM USG IN DIFFICULT SITUATIONS

ISUOG Practice Guidelines on intrapartum ultrasound suggested the following indications for ultrasound in labor include slow progress or arrest of labor in the first stage or second stage, ascertainment of fetal head position and station before considering or performing instrumental vaginal delivery and an objective assessment of fetal head malpresentation.[3]

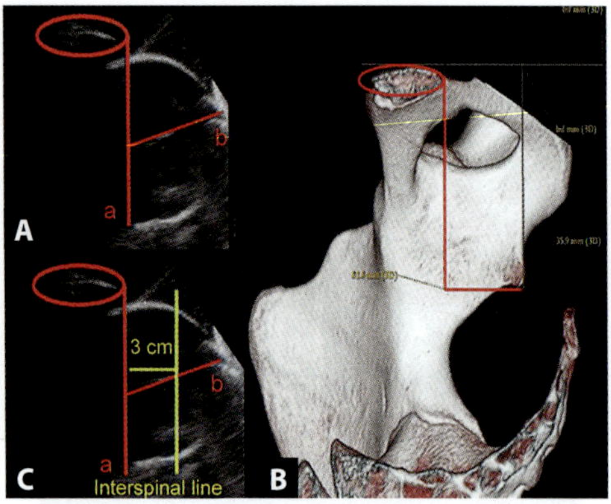

Fig. 8: Head station.

Fetuses with abnormal labor and occipito-posterior position had deflexed presentations in 14% of cases and were never delivered vaginally. Sonography was far more accurate than digital examination in such patients to decide earlier on for a cesarean section. A deeply impacted fetal head and a second-stage cesarean section is associated with increased maternal risks such as major hemorrhage, bladder injury, and extension tears of the uterine angle resulting in broad ligament hematoma. Such complications can be averted by early prediction using USG.[4]

The 2020 Royal College of Obstetricians and Gynaecologists assisted vaginal birth guideline recommends the use of intrapartum ultrasound for a fetal-head position where there is clinical doubt before applying an instrument. The degree of rotation, fetal-head station, and direction of the fetal head can help in reaffirming the decision to proceed with an assisted vaginal delivery or a cesarean section.[5]

CONCLUSION

In the ever-changing dynamics of the process of normal labor, precision in the diagnosis of abnormal patterns goes a long way in ensuring the safety of labor. The use of intrapartum ultrasound in the assessment of the progress of labor ushers in an objective and evidence-based method of determination. It is simple to learn, not time-consuming, and with consistent use, offers a colossal improvement in labor management. It is neither superior to digital examination nor must be thought of as a replacement. It must be used to correlate alongside clinical findings, to objectively reiterate the subjective examination. It finds special use in tricky situations like occipito-posterior or prolonged labor and avoids traumatic or failed instrumental deliveries.

REFERENCES

1. Armbrust R, Henrich W, Hinkson L, Grieser C, Siedentopf JP. Correlation of intrapartum translabial ultrasound parameters with computed tomographic

3D reconstruction of the female pelvis. J Perinat Med. 2016;44(5):567-71. doi: 10.1515/jpm-2015-0395.

2. Malvasi A, Stark M, Ghi T, Farine D, Guido M, Tinelli A. Intrapartum sonography for fetal head asynclitism and transverse position: sonographic signs and comparison of diagnostic performance between transvaginal and digital examination. J Matern Fetal Neonatal Med. 2012;25(5):508-12.
3. Barbera AF, Tinelli A, Malvasi A. Asynclitism: Clinical and Intrapartum Diagnosis in Labor. In: Malvasi A (Ed) Intrapartum Ultrasonography for Labor Management, 1st edition. 2013. pp.73-86.
4. Bellussi F, Ghi T, Youssef A, Cattaneo I, Salsi G, Simonazzi G, et al. Intrapartum ultrasound to differentiate flexion and deflexion in occipitoposterior rotation. Fetal Diagn Ther. 2017;42(4):249-56.
5. Archana A. Novel method to assess fetal head station in labour correlation between the clinical method of determination of fetal head station and transperineal ultrasound method of determination of fetal head station. IOSR Journal of Dental and Medical Sciences. 2018;17(2):1-4.

9

CHAPTER

Ultrasound Measurement of Cervical Length

Aditi Shastri

WHY?

An estimated 13.4 million babies were born preterm (PTB) in 2020. 55.6% of total livebirths are in Southern Asia and Sub-Saharan Africa, yet they accounted for 65% of the PTB.[1]

15% of deliveries prior to 34 weeks have history of PTB in the prior pregnancy (3% of the pregnant population) and the remaining 85% come from the 97% of pregnancies which are either first conceptions or those with prior term delivery.[2] Hence, treatment strategies have moved from history indicated treatment to ultrasound guided cervical length (CL) assessment in confirming threatened preterm labor (PTL)[3] and now universal screening for CL at various gestations in pregnancy in order to apply effective prevention strategies.

USG measurement of CL at term can help with optimizing timing and method of delivery. In women with need for planned cesarean sections, CL assessment at 37 weeks: when <20 mm, there is a 95% chance of spontaneous onset of labor before 40 weeks. While >30 mm there is a 95% chance that spontaneous onset of labor will not occur before 40 weeks.[4] Deliveries can be optimally timed accordingly.

Furthermore, in women undergoing induction of labor for post-dated pregnancies, CL helps in counseling and decision making by predicting induction to delivery interval and likelihood of vaginal delivery/cesarean section (Parous women having failure rates of 2% for CL of 1–10 mm to 20% for CL >30 mm. Nullipara 10% for CL of 1–10 mm to 70% for CL >30 mm).[5]

WHEN?

The CL is generally stable between 14–28 weeks of gestation and tends to shorten gradually afterwards.[6] Routine CL measurement during pregnancy has been implemented.

In some populations, with subsequent reductions in PTB rate and is supported by many national and international bodies,[7,8] as part of the second-trimester anomaly scan. Measurements taken prior to this tend to overestimate CL, due to the difficulty in identifying the internal os and incorporation of the underdeveloped lower uterine segment. 24 weeks is usually the upper limit for screening strategies, as preventive measures (progesterone/pessaries/cerclage placement) are usually withheld and therapeutic interventions (tocolysis, administration of antenatal corticosteroids) can be implemented.[7,9] Prepregnancy measurements of CL are not useful for predicting PTB in subsequent pregnancies.[10]

In asymptomatic women with previous history of PTB and in those with uterine abnormalities, such as unicornuate uterus, CL should be measured every two weeks at between 14 and 24 weeks of gestation and routinely at the time of the second trimester scan at 20–24 weeks when any such history is absent.[11]

Recent studies and metanalysis have established an association between first-trimester CL and risk of short cervix in the second trimester.[12] A cursory assessment of the CL is recommended during the first trimester scan if there are no cost or logistical constraints.

WHO?

Standardized protocol and sequential assessments are of the essence in optimal CL assessments. The aim of introducing ultrasound as a screening tool was to reduce the inter-/intraobserver variability. Hence, diligent training methods and correct understanding of the technique are of utmost importance in optimizing outcomes. Among the numerous available methods, The Fetal Medicine Foundation's Certificate of Competence in Cervical Assessment[11] and the Cervical Length Education and Review (CLEAR) Program[13] are the two high-standard Internet-based educational courses that award certification for professionals who complete the theoretical course and submit scan images for audit.

HOW?

Cervical measurement can be done by one of the three methods:[14]

1. **Transvaginal (Preferred):**

   Prerequisites

   - Counseling and willingness of the patient
   - Vaginal ultrasound transducer covered with disposable sheath (condom cover), lubricated with gel on both sides with caution to remove air bubbles
   - Dorsal lithotomy position
   - *Empty bladder:* Full bladder can increase artificially the cervical length and can obscure the presence of funneling by compressing the two halves of the funnel together. The mean difference between CL on empty bladder and that on full is about 4 mm.

Technique

- The ultrasound probe is introduced in the vagina and directed in the anterior fornix. Avoid exerting undue pressure on the cervix, which may artificially increase the length.
- The sagittal view of the cervix is obtained.
- Visualize inferior bladder border, external os, endocervical canal and mucosa (which may be of increased or reduced echogenicity compared to the cervix) which are a guide to the true position of the internal os and help avoiding confusion with the lower segment of the uterus.
- Minimize pressure and ensure that both cervical lips have same width, keeping all required structures in image
- Cervix should occupy 50–75% of screen.

Measurement

- Place calipers between functional internal os and external os, obtaining linear distance between the triangular area of echo density at the external os and the V-shaped notch at the internal os.
- If there is funneling, the caliper should be placed at the apex of the funnel.
- If the cervix exceeds 25 mm in length, it will be curved in more than 50% of cases. (Linear measurement will underestimate the cervical length in these cases). However, this is of little clinical significance as these patients are at low risk regardless of the exact measurement. *In the high-risk group of patients with a cervical length <16 mm, the cervix will always be a straight line.*
- In the first trimester, as the difference in CL between patients at risk of PTB versus those not is very small and hence a curved measurement may be taken for better distinction.
- Cervix being a dynamic structure, the examination should be done at least over a period of 3–5 min. Manual pressure at the fundus or asking patient to bear down may also be considered to assess dynamic shortening.
- *Reproducibility:* Difference between two measurements obtained by the same sonographer or by two different sonographers is about 4 mm.
- Obtain three distinct measurements. In about 1% of cases the cervical length may change due to uterine contractions. The shortest technically correct measurement should be recorded.

Assessment

- Thin cervical funnel needs to be differentiated from normal cervical mucus especially in the third trimester, which is best done by delineating the course of the fetal membranes: if they are not prolapsing into the cervical canal and are located at the level of the internal cervical os, the presence of a true funnel is unlikely. Funneling is *not* an independent risk factor for spontaneous PTL.

- A screen cut-off of 20 and 25 mm has been proposed by various studies with an increase in FPR from 1–4%. ISUOG proposes using a cut-off of 25 mm prior to 24 weeks as a '*Good Practice Point*' to initiate measures to prevent PTB in asymptomatic singletons and multiple pregnancies **(Fig. 1)**.[14]
- Other features to be identified:
  - Cervical sludge—independent risk factor for spontaneous PTB, preterm premature rupture of membranes (PPROM) and histological chorioamnionitis in asymptomatic patients
  - Vasa previa
  - Low-lying placenta—edge within 20 mm from the internal os **(Fig. 2)**

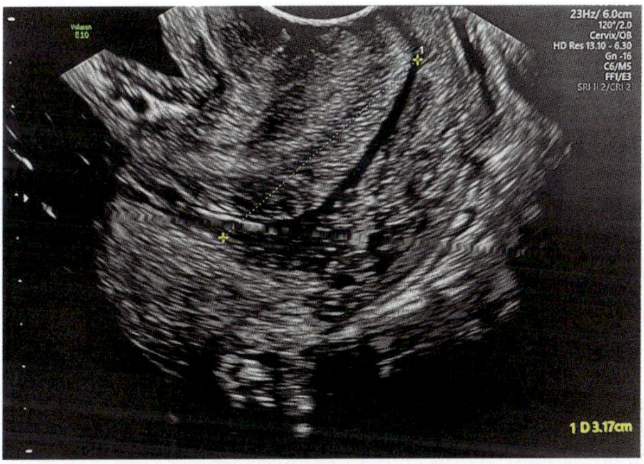

Fig. 1: Good practice point.

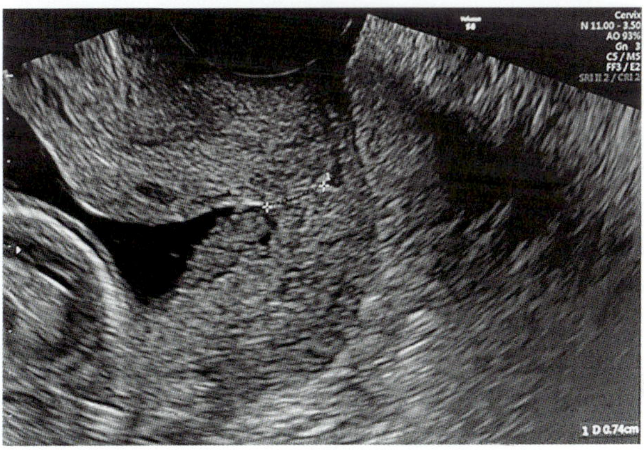

Fig. 2: Short cervix with funnelling and sludge.

2. **Transabdominal:** Restricted views, chances of overestimation due to full bladder. Can be used as an initial evaluation to be followed by proper approach.
3. **Transperineal:** Restricted use in cases of PPROM. Reduction in the detail in which the cervix is seen as probe is further away from the cervix. In 95% of cases, the difference between TVS and TPS measurements is within ± 5 mm.

WHAT'S NEW?

Cervical Shear Elastography

Elasticity of the cervix is determined based on motion in areas of the cervix compared to other areas outlined in the color map. The cervix is examined in the conventional way. Gentle pressure is then applied with the transducer to modify the tissue, and advanced software is used to create a color map that illustrates the deformation of the tissue compared to the nearby areas. Recent prospective studies and meta-analyses concluded that this is a promising method in predicting preterm birth and may even be superior to using cervical length alone.[15]

Cervical Consistency

This method involves measuring the ratio of the anterior to the posterior diameter of the cervix before and after exerting pressure on the cervix. This assumes that softer tissue changes more and has a lower cervical consistency index (CCI) than tougher tissue. The disadvantage is that there is no objective measure of force exerted prior to the calculation.[16]

Uterocervical Angle

A higher uterocervical angle (UCA) measurement (greater than 150°) is an important risk factor for deliveries before 37 weeks' gestation. Large meta-analyses do not give conclusive evidence towards the benefit of this method.[17]

WHAT'S MORE?

- In women with threatened PTL the rate of delivery within the subsequent 7 days is inversely related to cervical length at presentation. CL <20 mm (20% of threatened PTL and this group contains 75% of those that deliver within 7 days. CL >20 mm the risk of birth within 7 days is about 3%.[3]
- *Polyhydramnios:* Amnioreduction may precipitate preterm birth and is reserved for the cases where CL is <15 mm or serial scans demonstrate shortening to <25 mm.[11]

WHY NOT?

Despite applying universal screening and available preventive/therapeutic methods, there is only a marginal reduction of PTB in both the developing and developed nations alike given the poor understanding of the pathophysiology behind PTL onset and progression and lot more studies need to be done to optimize the same.

REFERENCES

1. Ohuma E, Moller A-B, Bradley E, et al. National, regional, and worldwide estimates of preterm birth in 2020, with trends from 2010: a systematic analysis. Lancet. 2023;402(10409):1261-71. doi:10.1016/S0140-6736(23)00878-4.
2. Celik E, To M, Gajewska K, Smith GC, Nicolaides KH; Fetal Medicine Foundation Second Trimester Screening Group. Cervical length and obstetric history predict spontaneous preterm birth: development and validation of a model to provide individualized risk assessment. Ultrasound Obstet Gynecol. 2008;31(5): 549-54. doi: 10.1002/uog.5333. PMID: 18432605.
3. Sotiriadis A, Papatheodorou S, Kavvadias A, Makrydimas G. Transvaginal cervical length measurement for prediction of preterm birth in women with threatened preterm labor: a meta-analysis. Ultrasound Obstet Gynecol. 2010;35:54-64.
4. Ramanathan G, Yu C, Osei E, Nicolaides KH. Ultrasound examination at 37 weeks' gestation in the prediction of pregnancy outcome: the value of cervical assessment. Ultrasound Obstet Gynecol. 2003;22:598-603.
5. Hilder L, Costeloe K, Thilaganathan B. Prolonged pregnancy: evaluating gestation-specific risks of fetal and infant mortality. Br J Obstet Gynaecol. 1998;105:169-73.
6. Iams JD, Goldenberg RL, Meis PJ, Mercer BM, Moawad A, Das A, et al. The Length of the Cervix and the Risk of Spontaneous Premature Delivery. N Engl J Med. 1996; 334: 567–73.
7. Society for Maternal-Fetal Medicine (SMFM). Electronic address: pubs@smfm, McIntosh J, Feltovich H, Berghella V, Manuck T. The role of routine cervical length screening in selected high- and low-risk women for preterm birth prevention. Am J Obstet Gynecol. 2016;215:B2–B7.
8. Di Renzo GC, Gratacos E, Kurtser M, Malone F, Nambiar S, Sierra N, et al. Good clinical practice advice: Prediction of preterm labor and preterm premature rupture of membranes. Int J Gynecol Obstet. 2019;144:340–46.
9. Berghella V, Talucci M, Desai A. Does transvaginal sonographic measurement of cervical length before 14 weeks predict preterm delivery in high-risk pregnancies? Ultrasound Obstet Gynecol 2003;21:140–44.
10. Ludmir J. Sonographic detection of cervical incompetence. Clin Obstet Gynecol. 1988;31:101–9.
11. The Fetal Medicine Foundation. Education. Cervical assessment. Internet based course. https://www.fetalmedicine.org/education/cervical-assessment.
12. Wulff CB, Rode L, Rosthøj S, Hoseth E, Petersen OB, Tabor A. Transvaginal sonographic cervical length in first and second trimesters in a low-risk population: a prospective study. Ultrasound Obstet Gynecol. 2018;51(5):604-13. doi: 10.1002/uog.17556. Epub 2018 Apr 2. PMID: 28639717.
13. Perinatal Quality Foundation. CLEAR. Cervical Length Education and Review. https://clear.perinatalquality.org.
14. ISUOG Practice Guidelines: role of ultrasound in the prediction of spontaneous preterm birth. Ultrasound Obstet Gynecol. 2022;60: 435–56.

15. Nguyen-Hoang L, Chaemsaithong P, Cheng YKY, Feng Q, Fung J, Duan H, Chong MKC, Leung TY, Poon LC. Longitudinal evaluation of cervical length and shear wave elastography in women with spontaneous preterm birth. Ultrasound Obstet Gynecol. 2024;63(6):789-97. doi: 10.1002/uog.27614. PMID: 38354177.
16. Baños N, Murillo-Bravo C, Julià C, Migliorelli F, Perez-Moreno A, Ríos J, et al. Mid-trimester sonographic cervical consistency index to predict spontaneous preterm birth in a low-risk population. Ultrasound Obstet Gynecol. 2018;51(5):629-36. doi: 10.1002/uog.17482. Epub 2018 Apr 10. PMID: 28370687.
17. Goldstein MJ, Bailer JM, Gonzalez-Brown VM. Uterocervical angle in predicting spontaneous preterm birth: a systematic review and meta-analysis. AJOG Glob Rep. 2023;3(3):100240. doi: 10.1016/j.xagr.2023.100240. PMID: 37396342; PMCID: PMC10310481.

10

CHAPTER

Liquor Assessment During Antenatal Ultrasound

Karthik Senthilvel

INTRODUCTION

The amniotic fluid provides space for the fetus's growth and development. Its presence in optimal amounts is crucial for fetal well-being. Severely reduced or absent amniotic fluid may result in pulmonary hypoplasia, and increased amniotic fluid may result in premature preterm rupture of membranes, leading to neonatal mortality and morbidity.[1] This article will discuss the imaging quantifying methods, criteria for diagnosing reduced and increased amniotic fluid, pitfalls, causes, and further evaluation.

IMAGING QUANTIFYING METHODS

Two widely used methods are the deepest vertical pocket (DVP) and the amniotic fluid index (AFI). To measure the deepest vertical pocket, one has to swipe the whole uterus and select the deepest pocket without a fetal part, placenta, or umbilical cord in between. Probe has to be held perpendicular to the floor, and the calibers are placed from inner to inner of the amniotic membrane. The amniotic fluid index is preferred in singleton pregnancies beyond 20 weeks. To measure the amniotic fluid index, divide the uterus into four quadrants, measure the anterior-posterior diameter of the deepest pocket in each quadrant in centimeters, and consider the sum of all four, as shown in **Figure 1**. Pockets less than 1 cm should be excluded from the calculation. When no fluid pockets are measured 1 cm wide, it could be diagnosed as severe oligohydramnios with only a few pockets of fluid that cannot be measured. For the measurement of the deepest vertical pocket, the single largest pocket anywhere in the uterus is identified and measured as shown in **Figure 2**. It is preferred in multiple gestations and singleton gestations less than 20 weeks.[2]

CRITERIA FOR DIAGNOSING REDUCED AND INCREASED AMNIOTIC FLUID

Oligohydramnios is defined as a DVP measurement of less than 2 cm and an AFI of less than 5 cm. The complete absence of amniotic fluid is known

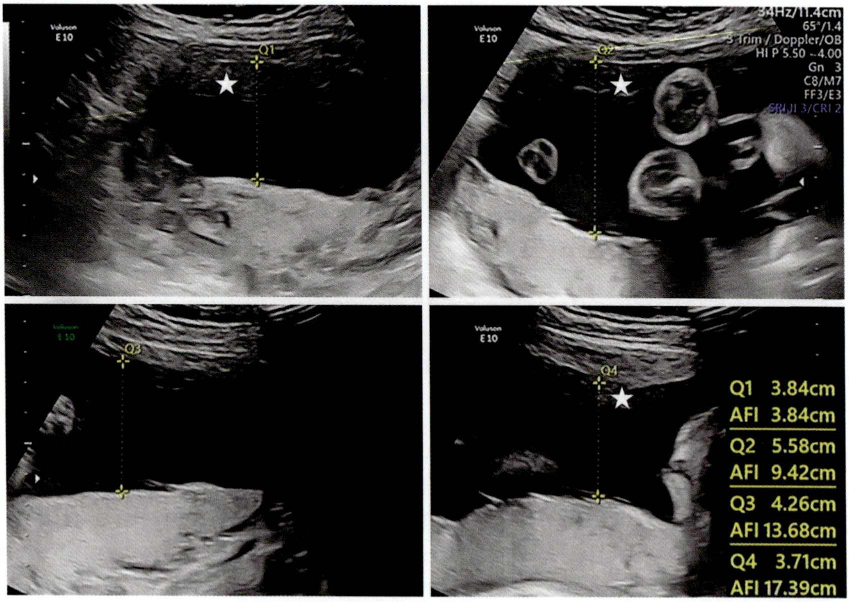

Fig. 1: Transabdominal grayscale image showing measurement of amniotic fluid index in a 28-week-old fetus. Star denotes the reverberation artifact near the anterior myometrium. Note the calibers being placed from the inner amniotic surface to the inner amniotic surface without any fetal part, placenta, or umbilical cord in between.

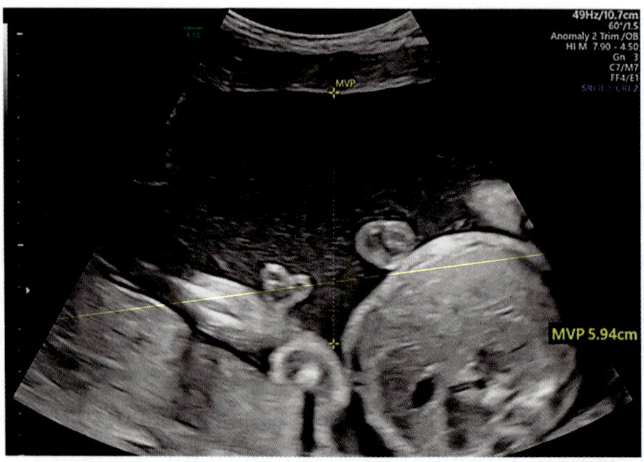

Fig. 2: Transabdominal grayscale image showing measurement of deep vertical pocket in a 28-week-old fetus. Note the calibers being placed from the inner amniotic surface to the inner amniotic surface without any fetal part, placenta, or umbilical cord in between. This can be even in the middle of the uterus.

as anhydramnios. Polyhydramnios is defined as a DVP of 8 cm or more or an AFI of 24 cm or more.[2] Current guidelines recommend using DVP to diagnose oligohydramnios and AFI to diagnose polyhydramnios, as AFI could overdiagnose oligohydramnios, and DVP could overdiagnose

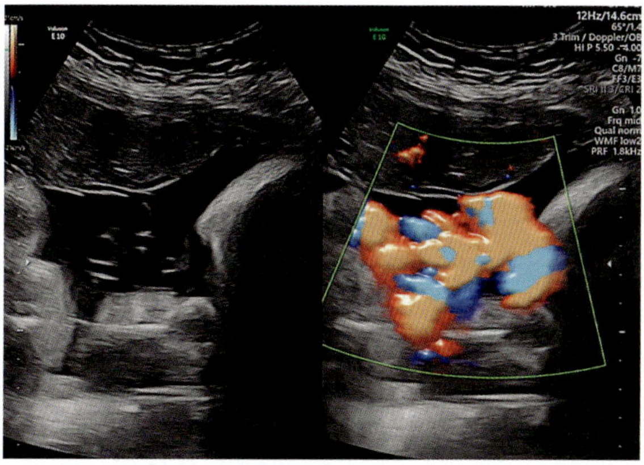

Fig. 3: Transabdominal grayscale and a color image showing an amniotic fluid pocket that is completely filled with umbilical cord but not so evident in grayscale.

polyhydramnios.[3-5] Amniotic fluid changes with gestational age, and gestational age-based nomograms are available. However, they are not widely used.

PITFALLS

- Reverberation artifact may mimic anterior myometrium as shown in **Figure 1**.
- In the maternal abdomen with poor penetration, a pocket filled with an umbilical cord may look anechoic and mimic an amniotic fluid pocket, as shown in **Figure 3**. Using color Doppler in such situations might be helpful.
- Umbilical cord cysts, cystic hygromas, and distended urinary bladder can be mistaken as amniotic fluid pockets.
- Far lateral approach might underestimate the amniotic fluid volume.

ASSESSMENT OF UNDERLYING ETIOLOGY

Oligohydramnios secondary to fetal genitourinary causes usually present between 13- and 21-weeks' gestation and ones due to placental or maternal causes presents between 34- and 40-weeks' gestation. Maternal causes include spontaneous or iatrogenic PPROM. Fetal causes include obstructive pathology such as posterior ureteral valve or functional causes such as autosomal recessive polycystic kidney disease or dysplastic kidney disease. Placental insufficiency can result in oligohydramnios and fetal growth restriction.

Polyhydramnios can result from maternal causes such as diabetes or fetal causes such as gastrointestinal atresia, neck masses, arthrogryposis akinesia sequence, and so on. Even placental masses like chorioangioma can cause polyhydramnios. Whenever the diagnosis of oligohydramnios or polyhydramnios is made, a detailed maternal history and ultrasound evaluation of the fetus and placenta must be done.

A recent literature review concluded that there is not enough evidence to suggest prenatal genetic testing with chromosomal microarray in cases of isolated oligohydramnios.[6] However, isolated polyhydramnios is shown to be associated with karyotype abnormalities.[7] Additionally, polyhydramnios with structural abnormalities is associated with several microdeletion and microduplication, so direct fetal testing can be considered.[8]

FETAL INTERVENTIONS

Interventions such as amnioinfusion or amnioreduction may be necessary for severe oligohydramnios or polyhydramnios, respectively. Amnioinfusion, the injection of sterile saline into the amniotic sac, helps in cases of severe oligohydramnios to support better visualization of fetal anatomy and lung development. Ongoing clinical trials are exploring the effectiveness of amnioinfusion in cases of anhydramnios with renal causes.[9] Conversely, amnioreduction is used in polyhydramnios to reduce amniotic fluid volume and relieve maternal discomfort. Amnioreduction is indicated for severe maternal discomfort, dyspnea, cervical length of less than 15 mm, or AFI of more than 35 cm. Complications are rare but may include chorioamnionitis and PPROM.[10]

CONCLUSION

Monitoring AF levels is essential for assessing fetal well-being, and any disturbances in amniotic fluid volume may indicate underlying issues requiring prompt intervention. Ultrasonography remains the gold standard for evaluating amniotic fluid volume, and understanding the causes and treatments for amniotic fluid abnormalities can significantly improve pregnancy outcomes.

REFERENCES

1. Dubil EA, Magann EF. Amniotic fluid as a vital sign for fetal wellbeing. Australas J Ultrasound Med. 2013;16(2):62-70. doi: 10.1002/j.2205-0140.2013.tb00167.x. Epub 2015 Dec 31. PMID: 28191176; PMCID: PMC5029989.
2. Jha P, Raghu P, Kennedy AM, et al. Assessment of amniotic fluid volume in pregnancy. Radiographics. 2023;43(6):e220146. doi:10.1148/rg.220146.
3. Hughes DS, Magann EF. Antenatal fetal surveillance assessment of the AFV. Best Pract Res Clin Obstet Gynaecol. 2017;38:12-23.
4. Dashe JS, Pressman EK, Hibbard JU; Society for Maternal-Fetal Medicine (SMFM). SMFM Consult Series #46: Evaluation and management of polyhydramnios. Am J Obstet Gynecol. 2018;219(4):B2–B8.

5. American Family Physician. Don't use amniotic fluid index to make a diagnosis of oligohydramnios (in the third trimester). https://www.aafp.org/ pubs/afp/ collections/choosing-wisely/414.html. Accessed March 21, 2023.
6. Singer A, Maya I, Sukenik-Halevy R, et al. Microarray findings in pregnancies with oligohydramnios: a retrospective cohort study and literature review. J Perinat Med. 2019;48(1):53-8. doi:10.1515/jpm-2019-0228.
7. Sagi-Dain L, Sagi S. Chromosomal aberrations in idiopathic polyhydramnios: a systematic review and meta-analysis. Eur J Med Genet. 2015;58(8):409-15. doi:10.1016/j.ejmg.2015.06.010.
8. Wu X, Li Y, Lin N, Su L, Xie X, Liang B, et al. Evaluation of genetic variants using chromosomal microarray analysis for fetuses with polyhydramnios. BMC Med Genomics. 2022;15(1):73. doi: 10.1186/s12920-022-01224-w. PMID: 35354480; PMCID: PMC8966299.
9. Atkinson MA, Jelin EB, Baschat A, et al. Design and Protocol of the Renal Anhydramnios Fetal Therapy (RAFT) Trial. Clin Ther 2022;44(8):1161-71.
10. Erfani H, Diaz-Rodriguez GE, Aalipour S, et al. Amnioreduction in cases of polyhydramnios: indications and outcomes in singleton pregnancies without fetal interventions. Eur J Obstet Gynecol Reprod Biol. 2019;241:126-128. doi:10.1016/j.ejogrb.2019.05.019.